Recipes for a
Better Menopause

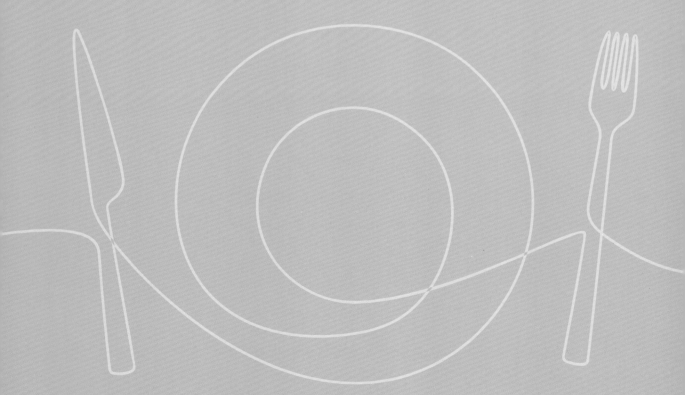

Recipes for a Better Menopause

A life-changing, positive approach to nutrition for pre, peri & post menopause

DR FEDERICA AMATI & JANE BAXTER

CONTENTS

Introduction
By Dr Federica Amati

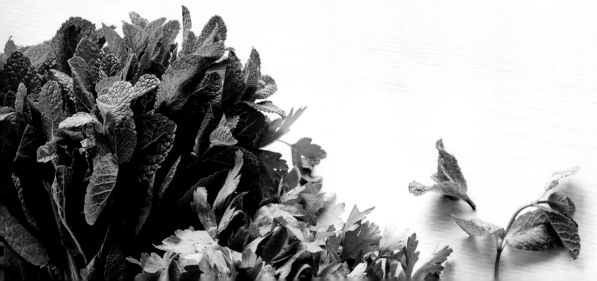

Recipes

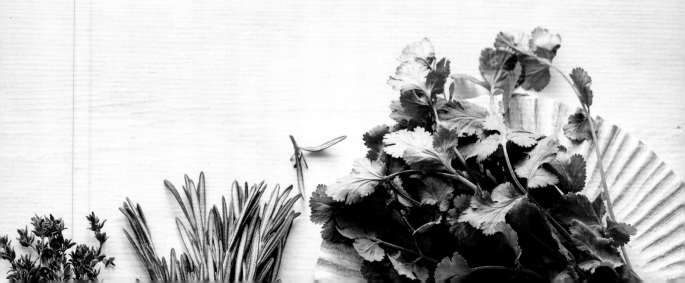

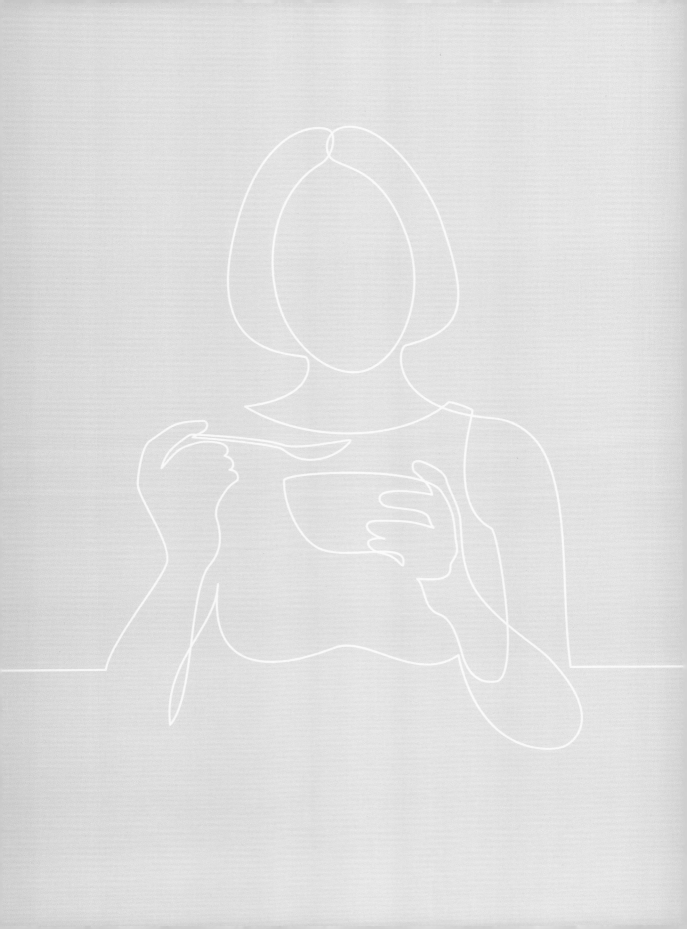

This is a book for all women and those who love them. The universal reality of menopause is that all women will go through it — whether premature, natural, surgical or later than average. History shows it has been under-researched and mistreated in medicine. Now we have enough momentum, research and interest for a more positive outlook. The knowledge we have, and how we can harness food to ensure our best possible long-term health, is exciting and empowering.

The good news is that by incorporating new scientific learnings into our diet, women can reduce the unfavourable health impacts of menopause during the transitionary period and beyond, either directly by reducing inflammation and excessive blood sugar spikes or indirectly by altering the gut microbiome. The recipes in this book taste delicious and draw on the latest research, introducing you to small dietary changes that will make a big difference to your health.

Dr Federica Amati

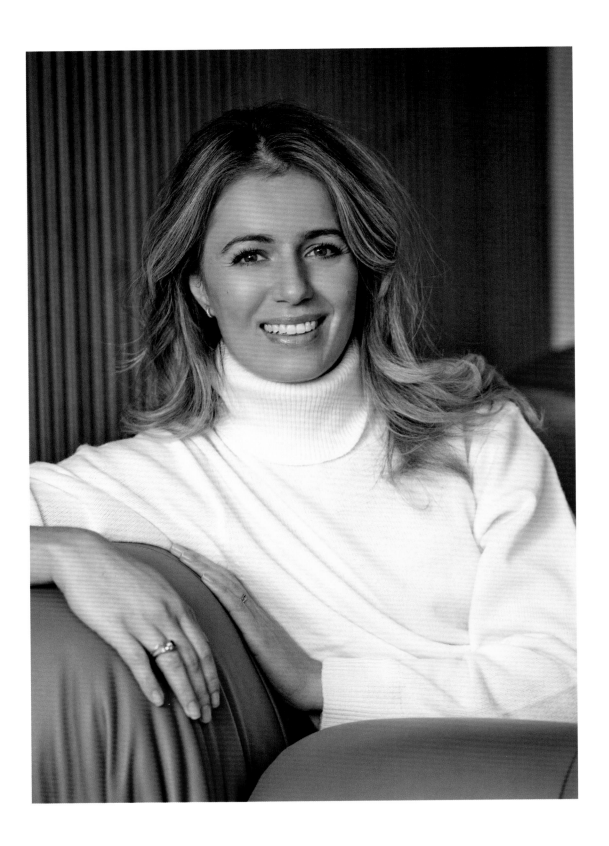

Introduction by Dr Federica Amati

Working across public health research and nutrition, I have always been struck by the pivotal impact that women's health has on the overall health of society. It's well established in research worldwide that empowering women, improving their access to good food and healthcare and ensuring they have the tools they need to thrive not only benefits the men, children and elders in their lives, but also contributes to economic growth and reduced violence. My own experience as a mother of two young children reinforces my understanding of this theory: if I don't look after myself, I can't look after my family. I vividly remember that when my mother underwent surgical menopause, our household ground to a halt as we adapted to life without our central cog for a while.

Working in PR and communications to fund my years of studying taught me how powerful clear and actionable messaging can be. I thought that if I could make evidence-based public health and nutrition information as engaging as the latest film industry event, the impact on people's health could be huge! Leading a double life of academia by day and luxury hospitality PR by night confused many of my friends and family, but these two very different skills eventually landed me my dream career. I am an academic and teach at one of the best universities in the world, have a busy nutrition clinic, work across science communications at ZOE (the personalized nutrition company running the world's largest nutrition-science study) and get the opportunity to write about science and nutrition every day for medical journals and press, as well as speaking on podcasts and at live events and conferences. I have always loved medical science and, from a young age, wanted to work with people to help improve their lives. Fast forward to 2018 and I found that writing about science and health, on topics covering nutrition and pregnancy, menopause, mental health and the microbiome could reach and help people in a way I had never thought possible as a young student.

I initially applied to be a medical doctor; the obvious career path for a doctor's daughter who wanted to help people. But the universe had other ideas and the day before my all-important chemistry exam, my beloved grandmother, who had been living with us for her final years, died of type 2 diabetes complications. I turned up to the exam and mostly stared into space, which funnily enough didn't result in the predicted A grade I needed to secure my university spot at Imperial College London. This first bump in the road was actually the beginning of my unorthodox path to becoming a public health nutritionist and academic instead. Ironically, I now teach nutrition to Imperial College medical students, which feels like a lovely way to complete that circle.

Over the many months of hospital work experience I undertook as a teenager, I saw that the doctors I followed were trained to efficiently manage patients with complex multimorbidities (multiple different long-term conditions all happening together). I, on the other hand, was concerned by the systems in place which led the patients to be in that situation. Entire wards of people were suffering from diseases that were much more easily prevented than cured, and I couldn't help but think that they could have avoided being there in the first place. Similarly, lots of the debilitating symptoms that people experience on a day-to-day basis (like sleep problems, constipation, low mood and anxiety) can often be prevented or improved by simple lifestyle changes, leading to drastic improvements in quality of life. My grandfather was the perfect example of this phenomenon. He had a heart attack and triple bypass after more than three decades of smoking and eating the wrong foods for his biology. Literally overnight, he changed his lifestyle and diet and not only made an incredible recovery, but also ended up teaching exercise classes to fellow heart attack survivors decades younger than himself. He even became the oldest person to run the Rome marathon in his eighties. During his final years, his positive attitude and thirst for life never left him. When he passed away in his late nineties, I knew that his final decades would never have been possible had he not made the changes to his diet and lifestyle which he did in midlife.

Instead of medicine, I went on to study biomedical sciences, where I could learn more about the fundamental science I loved, and then specialize with an honours in endocrine pharmacology. This was the first of many lightbulb moments. I was fascinated by the delicate balance of human hormones and health. It inspired me to study for a Masters in Public Health and a PhD in clinical medicine research, expand my public health and epidemiology skills and finally complete an MSc in nutrition as the tool to deliver the knowledge at an everyday level. My journey to becoming a nutritionist began when, as a postgraduate student, a lecture by Professor Elio Riboli, the principal investigator for EPIC, one of the world's largest studies on lifestyle and cancer, shifted my entire view on chronic disease[1]. He presented data from nearly half a million people all over Europe, and the associations that could be made between foods and diseases. From what Professor Riboli was telling us, our Western diets and lifestyles were causing an increase in many cancers across all age groups. Suddenly, I realized that the chronic diseases I associated with my elderly grandparents were present in my midlife father, whose sedentary lifestyle, lack of enthusiasm for fruits and vegetables and love of cured meats were putting him at risk. Looking back on it now, I often wonder if his premature death of colon cancer aged just 63 could have been prevented if he'd known about the impact that changing those habits could have had on his health and longevity.

> Diet can be our biggest ally for good health during menopause and beyond and the delicious recipes by Jane Baxter show us how we can make these foods part of our everyday eating routine.

Modern medicine and improved hygiene have helped us survive infectious diseases that in the 1900s would have killed so many of us, but our modern lifestyles and food environment are doing a good job of counteracting these improvements. Obesity rates have doubled since the 1980s and chronic diseases now cause the equivalent of 74% of all deaths globally, with smoking, physical inactivity and poor diet established as the main drivers[2]. This means nearly three out of four deaths all over the world are due to diseases we could prevent or delay with changes to our daily habits, often vaguely termed as 'lifestyle changes'. Menopausal women are no exception — in fact, it's quite the opposite. Chronic diseases affect more women than men, with post-menopausal women at highest risk (more on this later)[3]. The power lies in recognizing that these lifestyle changes are actually habits, and habits are formed; they are consciously adopted behaviours at first, which then become automatic second nature over time. This book looks at how our diet can be our biggest ally for good health during menopause and beyond, and the delicious recipes by Jane Baxter show us how we can make these foods part of our everyday eating routine.

Why women's health?

Women's health and improving quality of life is something that has been central to my work and research since my very first public health thesis, which focused on the importance of person-centred care[4]. Understanding an individual, their motivations and needs is something that the historically more paternalistic approach in medicine did not factor in. The doctor knew best, and patients were simply to follow instructions.

Research priorities followed a similar pattern, with women's symptoms (and women as a group) often excluded from research entirely up until 1993, with the short-sighted idea that this 'protected' women from harm. In reality, it led to almost no evidence on what works for our bodies.

Times have changed now and anyone in the health and medical professions knows that listening to people is one of the most important skills a person can have. Historically, almost every doctor was male, and everything from period pains to breastfeeding to mood disorders were considered either inevitable events or 'hysterical' (from the Greek word for uterus!) problems to be dealt with or not mentioned at all. Despite improvements in diagnosing women's pain, there is still a gender gap in treating women with the highest standard of care. A 2019 study looking at how improved specific blood tests for heart attacks resulted in more women receiving the correct diagnosis (a 42% increase in heart attack diagnosis in women), but there was a still a huge discrepancy in treatment and outcome, with women still receiving only half of the appropriate treatments compared with men[5].

Diagnosing perimenopausal symptoms requires listening and never dismissing women's intuition and knowledge of themselves. Often women will describe their symptoms to me in clinic, excusing themselves as they do so. 'I don't feel like myself at the moment, but I guess that's normal for a lot of us,' or, 'I don't think I've changed my diet much, but I am heavier than I've ever been so I must be doing something wrong,' and even, 'I feel like I'm not very good at my job anymore so perhaps it's best if I quit.' With a little bit of time and opportunity for insight, the picture becomes clearer, and women realize that they aren't losing touch with reality; their reality is changing. There is often a powerful 'aha' moment when women discover the reason for their changing physical and mental symptoms and are offered a plan to help. On a couple of occasions, though, my clients have been so shocked to think that they might be perimenopausal from the symptoms they're presenting with, that they've chosen to investigate with more testing of their hormones or other metrics. It's important to remember that hormone tests can't diagnose perimenopause alone. While a hormone test can tell you if you're menopausal, perimenopause comes with such huge variations in hormones throughout a day, week or month that each hormone test is just a snapshot of a rollercoaster. Like a jigsaw puzzle, you'd need to take dozens of snapshots to try and figure out whether you're travelling up, down, looping round, backward or forward! A woman's own story of changing symptoms is the best insight.

Specializing in women's health was a natural choice for me as I entered the realms of confusion and misinformation when pregnant with our first baby. The obvious lack of clear, evidence-based and actionable advice for pregnant women or those trying to conceive shocked me. I began doing my own research and collating the evidence into a blog which I shared with friends when they asked for advice. I gathered data from different studies and presented the information as clearly as possible to

> **While a hormone test can tell you if you're menopausal, perimenopause comes with such huge variations in hormones throughout a day, week or month that each hormone test is just a snapshot of a rollercoaster.**

allow anyone to make their own evidence-based decision. That blog eventually led me to publish a review on the impact of the Mediterranean Diet on mothers' and babies' health (in short, the Med Diet is associated with better outcomes for mother and baby regarding everything from mental health to diabetes risk, allergies and even behavioural disorders). It was published in an international scientific journal[6] and still one of my most cited papers.

As a research scientist, I have witnessed how scientific findings can have significant impact when misapplied. One such instance is the false link established between the MMR vaccine and autism, which resulted in the study's author being struck off the UK medical register for scientific misconduct. Another less malicious example is the previous recommendation to avoid allergens such as peanuts during pregnancy to prevent allergies, which was later found to increase the likelihood of developing allergies. Hormone replacement therapy (HRT) for menopausal women is yet another example of how science can be misconstrued and lead to false conclusions. It was made all but impossible to prescribe HRT because of a study that showed an increased risk of breast cancer in the women who took it. However, the study participants had an average age of 60, which was approximately ten years post-menopause, and the type of hormone therapy they were given in the study is no longer the one used in clinical practice. For decades, the fear of breast cancer drove millions of women to not seek HRT, and many doctors avoided prescribing it until fairly recently.

Dr Sam Brown is a wonderful menopause specialist GP I have the pleasure of working with. As she explains, HRT is one of the options available for menopausal women and the risks and benefits are highly individual.

Hormone replacement therapy (HRT)
– Dr Sam Brown

DIAGNOSING MENOPAUSE

A question I'm often asked by women who come to my private and NHS menopause clinic is, 'How do I know when I am perimenopausal?'

It's easy to put menopausal symptoms down to other things, such as stress from work or relationships, caring for elderly parents or supporting children. At this time of life, we are often juggling a lot!

Please do take some time to talk to your doctor if you are not feeling quite yourself. They should be able to diagnose menopause based on your age, symptoms and by asking what is happening with your periods. It is very unlikely that you will need blood tests.

Hormones can fluctuate during perimenopause, so blood hormone levels are not always reliable. NICE (National Institute of Clinical Excellence) guidance advises doctors not to arrange blood tests for those above the age of 45 with typical symptoms. If you are younger than this, you can discuss with your GP or menopause specialist whether testing is right for you.

Blood tests can be done to rule out other things if needed – but be careful not to get caught up with complex, expensive and frequent blood testing. This really isn't needed.

WHAT IS HRT?

Hormone Replacement Therapy (HRT) treats the underlying cause of menopausal symptoms, by replacing the hormones that your body might need but is no longer producing. If you do decide to take HRT, then this is always best done in combination with a review of your lifestyle, looking at diet, exercise, sleep and stress management.

Although only one in ten women take HRT around menopause, for most women, the benefits outweigh the risks. HRT is effective at treating menopausal symptoms such as hot flushes, irritability, palpitations, tiredness, poor sleep, brain fog, low libido and vaginal dryness. HRT can also help protect bones against osteoporosis and reduce the risk of cardiovascular disease when taken within ten years of your last period. It is important that we raise awareness of the advantages of HRT as well as the risks, so that women who may benefit and want to take HRT can be fully armed with the facts.

You can take oestrogen-only HRT if you have had a hysterectomy, but you will need both oestrogen and progesterone if you have a womb. HRT can be given in different ways. It can seem confusing at first, but your doctor will be able to explain the best options for your stage of menopause.

Oestrogen
The safest way to take oestrogen is through the skin as a gel, patch or spray. This is a body-identical hormone, which means it has the same structure as the oestrogen made by your body.

Progesterone
Progesterone is required to protect the womb lining from being stimulated by oestrogen if you still have a womb. This can be taken as a body-identical

progesterone tablet (which is called Utrogestan in the UK) or as the Mirena coil, which can be inserted by a doctor into your womb. The Mirena coil can then also be used for contraception and heavy periods.

Doctors can also prescribe synthetic progesterone in a patch or tablet but this is less commonly prescribed now due to the availability of safer options.

Vaginal oestrogen

Oestrogen can also be taken vaginally, and this is a very safe way to treat vaginal dryness. Using vaginal oestrogen can also help with urinary symptoms, which can bother women at this time of life. This can be used on its own or alongside other methods of HRT.

Testosterone

Once you have established an HRT regime that suits you, it may be that you are still suffering from low libido, in which case testosterone can sometimes be helpful once other causes for this have been ruled out. This may be especially helpful for women who have premature ovarian insufficiency (POI) or who go through a surgical menopause. Testosterone can be given as a gel, which is absorbed through the skin.

Dose

The dose of HRT needs be personalized to each woman and her symptoms. It can take some time to feel better and the dose of HRT needed can also vary over time. It is important to track your symptoms and, if necessary, alter your HRT dose. Make sure you are having regular checks with your GP or menopause specialist to get your levels right.

Side effects

Side effects from HRT can include breast tenderness, bloating and water retention, and sometimes irregular bleeding when you first start. Some women are very sensitive to the progesterone, which can cause mood swings, irritability and bloating. Side effects usually settle – but if you continue to have side effects to progesterone, then there are ways of managing this.

MYTHS ABOUT HRT

HRT causes breast cancer
The risks of breast cancer with HRT have previously been overstated[7], but it is important to be breast aware. Always check your breasts for any changes and attend breast screening appointments when you are called for them.

The background risk of breast cancer for 1,000 women over a five-year period after the age of 50 is 23 per 1,000 women. This increases to 27 per 1,000 women if you take combined HRT (oestrogen and progesterone). But if your body mass index is over 30, then this would increase to 46 per 1,000 women. The infographic made by Women's Health Concern shows how these risks compare[8].

HRT delays the inevitable
HRT is used to ease symptoms during the transition to menopause. It does not delay the onset of menopause but can help women improve their quality of life and wellbeing while they have symptoms. If or when you decide to stop HRT, you can do this slowly to stop symptoms returning.

HRT causes blood clots
The newer types of HRT, which are given through the skin as a patch, gel or spray (transdermal) are not thought to be linked with any risk of blood

clots. There is no additional risk of blood clots with Utrogestan (the body-identical progesterone) either. Oral oestrogen is associated with blood clots and should not be taken if you have risk factors for blood clots, such as smoking.

You can only have HRT for five years

Lots of women believe that they can have HRT for five years only, and they may have been told this by their doctor. Some will then wait to start taking HRT until they are feeling very unwell with menopausal symptoms. It is important to know that there is no set time limit on treatment and that this is an individual decision.

If you are on HRT, always plan an annual check to confirm that the benefits outweigh the risks for you, and to ensure that the dose is correct. Your doctor can also discuss any new research data that has been established. Some women will be on HRT for the rest of their lives and feel much better for it.

HRT causes weight gain

Weight gain around the time of menopause is related to many factors, as is so well explained in this book. There is no conclusive evidence that HRT causes weight gain.

ALTERNATIVES TO HRT

If you do not want to take HRT, or if you can't take HRT due to a personal history of breast cancer, then there are lots of other options that you can try to reduce menopausal symptoms. Optimizing your diet, exercise pattern, sleep and stress levels are key. Alongside this you can also try:

1. **SSRIs (selective serotonin reuptake inhibitors)**
   Some types of antidepressants can be given, such as Citalopram or Venlafaxine. These can help to reduce hot flushes in some women.

2. **Oxybutynin**
   Oxybutynin has been shown to help hot flushes. It is usually prescribed for an overactive bladder.

3. **Gabapentin**
   This is a medication that is often used for epilepsy but there is some evidence that it can help with hot flushes, too.

4. **Neurokinin 3 receptor antagonists**
   This is a new drug that has been developed for the treatment of hot flushes in women who cannot take hormones.

5. **Vaginal moisturisers and lubricants**
   These can be helpful for vaginal dryness and are non-hormonal. It is important to choose ones that match the natural pH of the vagina. I usually recommend the Yes range of vaginal moisturisers and lubricants.

6. **Cognitive Behavioural Therapy (CBT)**
   This can be very effective for women both to reduce hot flushes and also to cope with the mood changes that can happen around

menopause. CBT is a talking therapy that focuses on how our thoughts, feelings and behaviour interact, and can help us with coping mechanisms to use when we are struggling.

7. **Mindfulness**

Mindfulness has been shown to help hot flushes, depression, anxiety and insomnia during menopause.

8. **Herbal medications**

Scientific evidence on herbal medicine effectiveness is lacking, but some women can find this helpful. You should discuss which ones might be best for you with your doctor as they can have side effects and interact with other medication. Always check that they have Traditional Herbal Registration (THR) marking on the packaging before buying new products.

Understanding the science

As this book is all based on scientific evidence, it's worth taking a moment to go through how science 'works'. Scientists fall largely into three simplified categories. First, there are laboratory scientists who run experiments in lab coats, have strict rules and processes for every single step and have to record everything that happens in the lab to make sure the experiment is reproducible by someone else. These scientists are the ones who can analyze and manipulate cells and find out about how drugs work at a cellular level. This is science that forms the foundation for a lot of what we know about health and disease today, but it is only part of the picture. A lot of studies at cellular level published by these scientists are taken as proof of effects in humans. This is a huge and problematic jump to make. Just because a chemical or drug or food makes a dramatic difference to cells *in vitro* (in a lab culture) does not automatically mean the same effect will be seen *in vivo* (in a live animal). It may do nothing at all, something completely different or could even be harmful because there are hundreds of processes that take place to carry that drug/ food from mouth to cell. That is why *in vivo* studies are always needed and often end up being published in scientific journals.

Animal studies follow when a plausible explanation of how something works is announced by lab results. Scientists can investigate how that possible effect seen *in vitro* (in cells) translates into mice, rats and house flies, for example. This is where the magic happens for a lot of nutrition and microbiome science as we can control these animals' environments in a way that we can't for humans. For example, it was thanks to an experiment in germ-free mice (born and bred without any microbes so that they are essentially a blank canvas to introduce gut microbes to) that scientists discovered the direct impact which the gut microbiome has on depression[9]. It's thanks to the *in vivo* animal studies that we now know that a change in gut microbiome can cause depressive behaviours in mice. Often these complementary *in vitro* and *in vivo* results are reported together to provide the full picture.

The second group of scientists work on answering human-related questions. Human studies are more complicated to run and more complex to interpret because it's impossible to keep people in the same environment for very long periods. This means that human studies are usually either short-lived, such as in a randomized controlled trial, or they have to account for many factors that impact people over time. These factors are individual, such as age, sex and ethnicity, lifestyle habits like alcohol consumption, use of over-the-counter medicines or recreational drugs, and societal factors sometimes referred to as the 'social determinants of health'; these include things like education level, income, employment and healthcare. When human studies are looking to determine an impact

When it comes to making a decision that may actually influence your health, this is the highest level of evidence we have to work with.

of something, they have to account for these 'confounders', which can have a significant effect on the outcome you are trying to measure. For example, if you have very little access to healthcare, you are more likely to get sick compared to someone who has very good healthcare access, so this has to be taken into account when trying to determine the likelihood of becoming ill. The results from these studies are then published in scientific journals as *peer-reviewed* papers (meaning that another three–four scientists have reviewed the work and think it is scientifically rigorous enough to publish), presented at conferences and sometimes make their way into the mainstream media.

Scientists in the third group don't work directly with cells, animals or humans, and they rarely wear a lab coat. These scientists apply systematic methods of research, clearly defining the question they want answering, how and at what time point, and then collating all the best and most relevant evidence to find the answer. They may also analyze large databases that are available through routine data collection in the health service or that have been made available by other scientists who have collected data on animals or humans, to answer some new questions. Often these scientists will review all of the available studies on a specific topic by reading all of the high-quality scientific studies available, analyzing the data and drawing a conclusion on what the published evidence shows so far. I am one of these third type of scientists. I have both analyzed large health data from populations with hundreds of thousands of data points, as well as reviewed other scientists' work to come to a conclusion on what we know on a topic *so far*. These are called systematic reviews and when there is enough original data to pool together, they can include a meta-analysis. To be able to conduct systematic reviews and meta-analyses there need to be enough *high-quality* studies to warrant reviewing them together to inform what effect A is having on B. When making a decision that may actually impact your health, this is the highest level of evidence we have to work with. Depending on the question you're asking, the type of study is very important. For example, if the question is about long-term associations, observational studies are best. Is drinking coffee associated with good health? Yes, according to observational data spanning over 30 years. But if you're looking to answer a question about how a specific thing has an impact on a specific outcome, for example: does everyone respond to a drug in the same way, a randomized controlled trial (RCT) is the right study. In some cases, such as in drug trials, large-scale RCTs hold more answers than a meta-analysis of observational studies.

Unfortunately, there are a lot of online 'health influencers' who take their experience of one person (themselves) to make recommendations on diet, lifestyle and even medication to very large audiences. A study of one person does not make scientific evidence; in fact, the rest of scientific media, including this book, video, social media post etc *is not scientific evidence*. If it is distributed with the intention of helping people with their health, it should be *evidence-based* and communicated clearly to make understanding the evidence easier for non-scientists (like this book!).

Hopefully this is helpful in understanding how scientific research works and what to look out for when people refer to evidence. The last thing to note is that if a piece of research is being paid for just by a private company or an industry, it is likely to preferentially report positive results. This is not as relevant for pharmaceutical trials (which are independently analyzed before regulatory approval) but is relevant to food-industry-funded studies. There are some astonishing examples of this, including a fizzy drink company famously pushing for studies on exercise to solve obesity in order to move the focus away from diet. Scientists have published findings that this kind of industry funding can skew results[10], so it's worth checking who funded a study.

Science vs menopause

Menopause is something that everyone born with ovaries will experience. We can choose to have children or not, or whether to take hormonal contraceptives which stop our menstrual cycles or not, but we will all experience menopause at some point. It is a shared experience — a fact that is both powerful and a great leveller. I am personally hugely motivated to look after myself differently since this realization. Since my ZOE test results showed that I already have poor blood sugar control now in my mid-thirties,

Scientific Evidence

Meta analyses and systematic reviews

Human trials and population studies

In vitro studies and animal trials

Case reports

Non-Scientific Evidence

YouTube videos, personal anecdotes, gut feelings, parental instincts, some guy you know, websites like Natural News, Info Wars, Natural Health Warriors, Collective Evolution, Green Med Info, Mercola.com, Whale.to, etc.

I have taken daily steps to help make sure I don't slowly inch my way towards type 2 diabetes. I know from my grandmother and now my mother that we have a genetic predisposition which accounts for roughly 40% of risk, and I also now know that menopause will accelerate any trend towards diabetes. Luckily, I have the tools to change direction and maximize my metabolic health with the food I eat and the ways I move my body daily, and feel strongly that all women should have their own tools to do the same.

Why and how does metabolism change during menopause? Does the gut microbiome play a part, or is it all down to ageing? Science still has a lot of questions to answer but we've made exciting progress in the past decade.

Women have started to share their menopause experiences and the tips and lifestyle changes which have helped them manage the symptoms, changes and challenges. There are examples of growth and liberation with this new chapter, as well as stories and statistics of women's lives being completely derailed; tens of thousands of women leave work because they're worried that they can't focus or perform well due to menopausal symptoms. Many of my clients speak about not recognizing themselves and not understanding why doing what they have always done no longer works for them physically, mentally and emotionally. Many women rejoice at never having to have a period again (85% of women in a 2022 poll!), or having to suffer from premenstrual symptoms or worry about unplanned pregnancy again. What was missing, alongside these personal stories, was solid scientific research to unpick these changes. Why and how does metabolism change during menopause? Does the gut microbiome play a part, or is it all down to ageing? Science still has a lot of questions to answer but we've made exciting progress in the past decade.

Medical research famously lacks women. Even in 2022, fewer than 25% of people in clinical trials for new drugs were women. This is a big problem, because more than half of us on this planet are female, and we do not always react to drugs, or food for that matter, in the same way as men. So why is there such a gap in data when it comes to women? Quite simply because we are more complicated to study. When recruiting women into a trial, researchers have to include an equal number of pre- and post-menopausal women (because they are so metabolically different, as we'll see later) and we also have to ensure we don't have any women who are pregnant or recently pregnant (again, because there is such huge physiological change around pregnancy). Basically, for every one man recruited into a study, we need to recruit at least two women, increasing the cost of these studies which are already difficult to fund.

Historically, women were not allowed to participate in clinical trials due to social restriction, but in the past 20 years the barriers have been mostly due to budgeting. The consequences are that we know less about female medical science than we do for males. The good news is that this is changing. Those who fund research have recognized the importance of including women, so more funds are being made available with women's inclusion as one of the caveats for fund eligibility. Large prospective cohort studies that aim to answer questions about long-term exposures and chronic diseases, such as EPIC, the Nurse's Health Study, and the ZOE Health study, include men and women alike.

I am lucky to work with a collection of wonderful people who are helping answer the important questions around women's health and menopause, using the evidence base available and filling the remaining research gaps. This includes menopause GP Dr Sam Brown and scientists Professor Sarah Berry and Dr Kate Bermingham, who are leading the world's largest menopause study. Professor Tim Spector investigated menopause during his PhD and leads the most exciting gut microbiome research, looking at improving healthy life span through gut health. Over the following pages, I'll talk you through the most up-to-date research which is leading to ground-breaking changes in the way we understand and manage menopause.

Menopause:
let's start at the beginning

Menopause is 'official' when a woman hasn't had a period for 12 months. For most women, this is around the age of 51, with 95% of women finishing their reproductive lives between the ages of 45 and 55. If menopause occurs before the age of 45, this is called early menopause, and before 40 it is called premature menopause, also known as premature ovarian insufficiency (POI). Premature menopause occurs in 1 in 100 women, with 1 in 1,000 before the age of 30. While for some women, premature menopause is caused by surgical or medical procedures (e.g., if you've had your ovaries removed), the majority (90%) of these women will have no known cause.

We know that genes contribute to nearly half (45%) of the variability in age of menopause onset[11]. This means that we inherit the age we enter menopause by quite a big margin. Other primates can reproduce throughout their lives for most of their lifespan, so the question of why humans evolved to end our reproductive lives earlier is one that scientists have tried to answer. One theory is that grandmothers play such a pivotal role in the health of their grandchildren, enhancing their survival and lifting some of the burden from their adult daughters, that it makes evolutionary sense to end reproductive age at a time when our first children are likely to be having their own children. Scientists who studied this in detail[12] found that the most important evolutionary drivers for a midlife menopause are the dramatic increase in maternal mortality for older mothers, and a benefit to grandchildren provided by the maternal grandmother. The best evidence points to grandmothers promoting grandchild wellbeing and enhancing their daughter's fertility (by reducing the childcaring burden thus reducing stress and a more rapid return to fertility), which is why this 'grandmother theory' of menopause onset has become my favourite. It is an important reminder of the crucial role that maternal grandmothers (or other mother figures) play in the evolution of our species.

Does what age you enter menopause matter?

Why is the age of menopause important for health? Aside from the fact that it dictates the end of our reproductive lives — some women find out they are perimenopausal when they are trying to conceive — it is also well established as a risk factor for our health. There are two main health conditions which are proven to be increased post-menopause: osteoporosis (weakened bones) and cardiovascular disease (heart and blood vessels). This is because oestrogen (one of the primary female sex hormones which controls our periods but also helps bone and heart function) rapidly declines post-menopause. Consequently, women who experience earlier menopause have more years with lower oestrogen levels, and so are at higher risk of developing these problems.

A systematic review and meta-analysis of nearly 200,000 women[13] found that early onset of menopause significantly increases the risk of type 2 diabetes by 15–50%, depending on how early you become menopausal, which is in turn associated with increased risk of cardiovascular disease. A pooled analysis of over 300,000 women[14] found that the risk of having heart disease before age 60 was almost twice as large for women who had premature menopause (before 40) and 1.5 times as large for those who entered menopause early (aged 40–44). These findings are controlled for other risk factors such as smoking and being overweight, so we know they're due to the earlier age of menopause.

We know that losing our oestrogen levels earlier than average is a problem, and women who become menopausal earlier than 45 should be monitored and supported swiftly and decisively to help prevent chronic health conditions. The earlier menopause happens, the more critical it is to get good support and guidance for long-term health. Early menopause is not that rare, and I've seen in my own clinic that women are often shocked when I suggest they may be perimenopausal in their early forties. Perimenopause itself can last up to ten years, with symptoms fluctuating throughout that time. Women in their early forties often dismiss their symptoms

Women in their early forties often dismiss their symptoms as being part of having a busy lifestyle, career, parenting or caring responsibilities, or all of these factors combined.

as being part of having a busy lifestyle, career, parenting or caring responsibilities, or all of these factors combined.

Overall, the average age of menopause has actually increased in the past 60 years[15] from 49 years old to 51 years old, and there has also been a decrease in the age at which women start their periods. This means our reproductive life spans have, on average, increased, but alongside this change there has also been an increase in hormonal disorders such as polycystic ovarian syndrome (PCOS)[16] and unexplained infertility. There are lots of factors that have contributed to these changes which include genetics, environment, access to healthcare and nutrition, and there are some brilliant scientists dedicating their research expertise to understanding some of the mechanisms at play. What's interesting to see is how younger women are much more interested and open about understanding their menstrual cycle and life cycle, in ways that my generation and my mother's certainly weren't.

This combination of a new interest in women's health, and more female scientists leading on that research, puts us at an exciting point in science history. In my own experience, I have seen the hugely beneficial impact that understanding our bodies and ourselves can have on our health. This is from my younger adolescent clients I have worked with to improve their nutrition, to couples I have supported along their fertility journey, to pregnant mothers I've supported through growing their babies and feeding them, to the wonderful women I have worked with through their perimenopause and their post-menopause health. One constant is that understanding ourselves as individuals with very unique responses to our hormones, our cycles, our food, our response to stress and our bodies is always the first step.

DOES WHAT YOU EAT IMPACT THE AGE OF MENOPAUSE?

The UK Women's Cohort Study (UKWCS) followed over 14,000 women and linked their diet with age of menopause, concluding that diets high in oily fish and legumes (hallmarks of the Mediterranean Diet) are more likely to have a later age of onset of menopause by three years compared with those women who ate lots of white rice and refined carbohydrates[17]. Weight, predominantly your adiposity level (amount of fat), also has a significant impact on age of menopause[18]. Women who are underweight are much more likely to experience early menopause, and those who are overweight experience the opposite.

It's worth noting that delaying menopause may also not be beneficial. Later age of menopause increases the risk of oestrogen-dependent cancers – endometrial, womb, breast and ovarian cancer – as does obesity. From what we currently know, there really does seem to be a sweet spot between 49 and 52 years of age for an ideal natural menopause onset. So is there a diet that can help to support us and our hormone health and avoid rushing or delaying the natural onset? Other factors such as genetics, when we had our first period, hormone disorders, medications, illness and other elements will also influence this timeframe. While changing genes is not very straightforward, making the right daily food choices can have a huge impact on our health and our gut microbiome, which is why I think nutrition is one of our greatest tools.

> A diet rich in vegetables, fruits and fibre was associated with a reduced risk of lung cancer, whereas a diet rich in red and processed meat was associated with an increased risk.

MENOPAUSE, NUTRITION AND THE BIG C

Breast cancer deaths have been steadily decreasing thanks to improved early diagnosis and treatment, but breast cancer cases have been steadily increasing at the same time. It will affect as many as one in eight women in high-income countries like the UK and the US and is the leading cause of ill-health in women. Some risk factors are caused by genetic changes, but the biggest increases in risk are seen due to modifiable factors. In a review of the risks in *Nature*[19], one of the best scientific journals in the world, the simplest ways to reduce breast cancer risk are to reduce obesity in post-menopausal women, reduce alcohol consumption to under two drinks per day, increase exercise and encourage women to breastfeed for 12 months or more in their lifetime.

Of interest for younger women is that the younger you have your first child, specifically before age 35, and the more children you have, the lower your risk. This is arguably not a modifiable risk factor, as having a child is highly dependent on many other factors but it's something which we as a society should be supporting women to do if they wish to start a family. Modern trends are exactly the opposite of this, and I work with lots of women who are struggling with their fertility in their late thirties and early forties, who often say to me that they wish they had known more about the science behind hormones, fertility, menopause and age earlier in their lives.

Combined oral contraceptive use and long-term menopausal hormone therapy (MHT) use are also associated with an increased risk of breast cancer, but it's worth noting that some of the benefits of these therapies, especially MHT, may outweigh the risk for many women. Other non-modifiable risk factors of predisposing genes (such as BRCA1 and CHEK2) and dense breast tissue are something to discuss with your doctor if you are worried.

What about other cancers? Looking specifically at women's risk in the second half of life, lung cancer, bowel cancer and womb cancer risk also increase with age. Womb cancer, like breast cancer, is often associated with oestrogen exposure, so women who have a late menopause or early menarche (first period) have an increased risk of this type of cancer, as do women who take hormone therapies for prolonged periods of time. Lung cancer, as we all know, is closely linked with smoking, pollution and inhaling toxic fumes through work or inside homes. Our diet can protect us from lung cancer too. A large study of over 400,000 people in the UK showed that a diet rich in vegetables, fruits and fibre was associated with a reduced risk of lung cancer, whereas a diet rich in red and processed meat was associated with an increased risk.

Colon cancer is the one where food choices make a huge impact. My beloved father passed away from colon cancer aged 63, so it's a subject close to my heart. A huge umbrella review of 45 meta-analyses, including 794 studies of hundreds of thousands of people, concluded that there is strong evidence that heavy alcohol intake (more than four drinks per day) and higher red meat consumption are associated with a significantly increased risk of bowel cancer. Even moderate regular drinking (say, a drink four nights per week) has a negative impact compared to occasional drinking or sobriety. On the flipside, higher fibre intake, calcium in the diet (found in all leafy greens) and yogurt intake (rich in probiotics) are all associated with a reduced risk of bowel cancer. These are clear associations, based on the highest quality evidence analysis so far. If, like me, bowel cancer runs in your family, you might reconsider alcohol and red meat intake and add plenty of leafy greens to your diet. We'll talk about natural yogurt and other probiotic foods for good gut microbiome health later in the book.

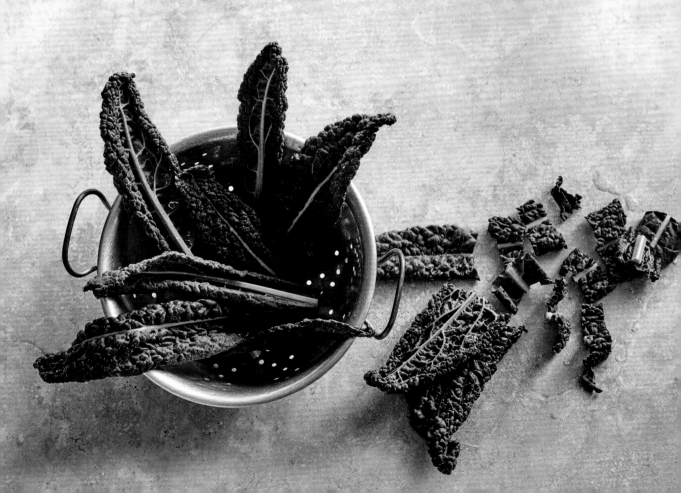

Preparing for menopause

Many women dread menopause and don't want to think about it until they have to. I have seen women who present at my clinic with perimenopausal symptoms and, as soon as I suggest they may be entering perimenopause, are visibly shocked at the suggestion. Of course, many menopausal symptoms are also signs of other conditions and we shouldn't fall into the trap of 'blaming menopause' for debilitating symptoms. Every woman needs to be assessed as an individual and every severe symptom thoroughly investigated.

I have had the privilege of researching and learning so much over the years about hormones, metabolism, medical science and nutrition from some of the most inspiring and respected scientists in their fields. And all of the knowledge I have gathered over this time has made me a real optimist about ageing and the power of prevention. We are at a pivotal point in scientific research, medicine and nutrition; there are now enough traditional and modern methods available that the number of tools we have to improve our health outnumbers the threats out there to damage it. This is not exclusive to those who are in their thirties; it is literally never too late to start improving the health of your future self. If we consider our health as an investment, there are no better returns than the ones we see on an investment in our health. As we'll see in more detail later in the book, introducing small changes as late as your nineties can significantly improve your health outcomes.

My diet has evolved so much over my lifetime. I vividly remember family meals in my Italian home (a non-negotiable) that involved pasta, vegetables, meat, fish and extra virgin olive oil in vast quantities. At university I often cooked for my flatmates and food for me had to be delicious, not just easy to make. In my early twenties I was lucky, through my work in hospitality and travelling around the world, to eat at some amazing restaurants. But my body didn't like all food equally and I noticed that I felt better when I ate less meat. I eventually became vegan in my twenties because I couldn't stomach the ethics of meat production and slaughter and found ways of making delicious food that also contained all the nutrients I needed with plants. Veganism is not for the time-poor or faint-hearted, though, and I ended up re-introducing oily fish and eggs, as well as traditional hard cheeses like Pecorino, to my diet when I became pregnant for the first time. Another pivotal moment in my life came when I lost that pregnancy and started using my academic skills to try to find answers, and frankly to distract myself from the loss. The changes to my diet then were all based on what I learned was needed for our bodies to make new life and, as I mentioned earlier, mothers' nutrition became an active area of research interest for me.

THE RHYTHM OF THE NIGHT: NUTRITION AND CIRCADIAN RHYTHM

Food can form the foundation of our future selves. The science of ageing is evolving, and we are getting many more insights into how what we eat and when we eat it can help us stay strong, sharp and spritely well into our older age. My understanding of the daily (aka circadian) rhythms of life has played a huge part in finding ways to juggle eating well with a busy work life and young children who love waking up very early all the time. Simply changing when we eat, without changing what we eat, can have the most profound effect on our biology. This is sometimes referred to as time restricted eating (TRE), a form of intermittent fasting. I like to think of it as sensible eating in response to our bodies, our schedule and our instincts.

Tuning in to the daily rhythms of when we wake, when we are most active and when we go to sleep can help us eat when we are supposed to, and rest when we are supposed to.

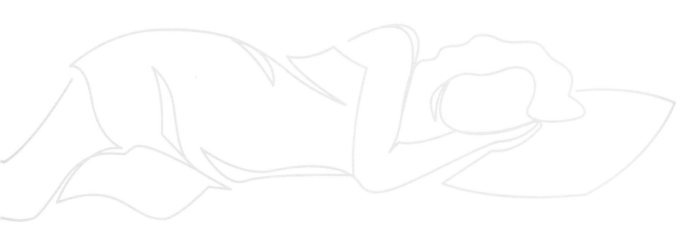

That sounds simple but it requires us to trust our own wisdom, which many of my clients have lost touch with over years of diets and following 'advice' such as 'kick start your metabolism with breakfast' and 'drink a glass of water if you feel hungry'. It can take a few weeks, but simply listening to your body's cues of hunger and fullness will often fall into a daily pattern. I'll use my own experience as an example: I used to eat breakfast before leaving the house

Tuning in to the daily rhythms of when we wake, when we are most active and when we go to sleep can help us eat when we are supposed to, and rest when we are supposed to.

without asking myself if I was hungry or not. It was just convenient for me to do this and then go to work. Equally, I would often feel ravenous by dinner time and eat lots of food right before going to bed, which often resulted in me going to bed later than I intended to because I just couldn't get to sleep on a full stomach.

Fast forward ten years and I have tuned in to my hunger cues like clockwork. I know I will be hungry for breakfast around 10am and will want to have dinner by 7pm. Most evenings I don't eat past 7pm and most mornings I don't eat before 9am. That means that for me, waking up on average at 6.30am and going to bed at 10.30pm, I have a 10-hour window in which I eat and a 14-hour window in which I drink water but don't really eat (unless, of course, I'm hungry). I make a conscious effort not to mindlessly graze on food (in my case most likely chocolate) between dinner and bedtime and instead I have my favourite chocolate at the end of my dinner. This seems simple enough, but I guarantee you it makes a marked difference because so many of us automatically eat when we are not hungry, both first thing in the morning and last thing at night.

The positive effect this approach to eating times has on our health is not because we are consuming fewer calories, but because we eat when our metabolism is ready to absorb and use food and we give our bodies the time to rest and repair overnight. Our gut microbiomes produce helpful microbes like Akkermansia, which activate when we are fasting (more on that later). We actually respond to our bodies' signals of hunger and fullness, which in turn improves those signal feedback mechanisms. Practising keeping in touch with my body's internal messaging systems and honouring the rhythm of the day and night is something I am sure will help me through my menopause transition as it is already helping me now.

Navigating the menopause maze: the interplay of stress, hormones and diet

Our hormone system is better known as the 'endocrine' system, which translates from the Greek for 'within secrete'. The tissues and organs involved in this signalling system essentially work by secreting either protein-based hormones (peptides, amines and proteins) or fat (lipid) hormones (including steroid, stress and sex hormones — e.g. oestrogen, progesterone and testosterone).

A diet that will support our health is also one that will support our hormones. Hormones are in delicate balance with the rest of our biology, continuously responding to instructions and information about our environment and our mental state. At a very basic level, this is crucial for survival. The reason why stress can dramatically impact our cycles, our hormones and our ability to conceive is simply because it triggers a protective response: if there is an outside stress that is threatening us as women, biology dictates that it probably isn't a good time to focus on reproductive potential. By this logic, being malnourished (which includes being underweight as well as having obesity with a lack of nutrients) results in our bodies shutting down the reproductive system first. Pregnancy and menstruation are very demanding processes that can push our bodies to depletion, so it doesn't make sense to risk that if we are to survive.

In modern Western society these perceived dangers are not as short-lived as they are for foraging and hunter gatherer tribes, which more closely resemble our evolutionary past. Many of us are chronically stressed, with cortisol levels elevated for weeks and months on end and not just while dealing with a crisis. We are stressed by our emails and the news first thing in the morning until we go to bed (still stressed) at the end of the day. Many of us won't even know the damage this is doing to our health until we reach a point of burnout or suffer more acute physical symptoms.

One of the first things to get overlooked when we do suffer from stress is our diet. Exactly when our bodies need it most, we often forego nutritious food, whole plants and home-prepared meals as we try to create more time to deal with the stress. Needless to say, this is the opposite of what we should be doing. Whether stress is acute, such as with an infection or injury, or chronic, our bodies need access to a range of nutrients and amino acids to respond, repair and return to normal function. The hypothalamus-pituitary-adrenal (HPA) axis is the central control hub of our stress response, but the hypothalamus is also responsible for sending our ovaries the chemical message that leads to oestrogen production, ovulation and our periods. If the central control hub is too busy responding to stress, our periods can stop[20]. It may not be surprising to read at this point that stress is strongly associated with worse menopausal symptoms[21]. This 2021 study showed that women who had recently experienced a stressful life event such a bereavement, suffered with 21% worse

Knowledge is power and while there are some stressful events we cannot control, and stress is of course a natural part of life, there are things we can do and habits we can put in place to help our bodies mitigate the effects of excess stress and stop it from overwhelming us.

symptoms compared to those who had not experienced stress. Menopausal symptoms are intrinsically linked to fluctuating hormones, and hopefully it's now clear that stress is a powerful player when it comes to changing hormone levels.

Stress is so influential in controlling our hormones that it can literally cause oestrogen levels to decrease to the point of stopping our menstrual cycle altogether, in the absence of any other medical issue. Disruption to our hormone levels and menstrual cycle impacts our likelihood of reaching average age of menopause onset, and as mentioned earlier, losing our oestrogen levels earlier in life is likely to put us at risk of health conditions later on. Knowledge is power and while there are some stressful events we cannot control, and stress is of course a natural part of life, there are things we can do and habits we can put in place to help our bodies mitigate the effects of excess stress and stop it from overwhelming us.

To help you build up your anti-stress toolkit, I have identified five main pillars of health that can help to reduce and mitigate the effects of excess stress: nourishment, movement, mindfulness, enjoyment and socializing. They exist together in many activities, so let's take a look at how to incorporate them into your daily routine and what the science tells us about each of them.

Nourishment – more than just food

Nourishment is a great word to describe the beneficial impact we get from eating nutritious food in a safe environment. It is more than eating and food alone. You can't get nourishment from a protein shake gulped in a rush on your morning commute. Science shows us that eating home-cooked food, which is freshly prepared and shared with those important to us is actually good for us[22], irrespective of what the dish is. Nourishment and socializing often, though not always, go hand in hand.

Whole books have been written on the importance of social structure and social function for health. Isolation is associated with increased risk of stroke, pneumonia and death[23] across a variety of countries and income levels. As our population structures continue to change, with predictions of a population rich in elderly people with fewer young people, we need to think ahead and begin creating a social structure that can increase our number of healthy, happy years of life.

Entering perimenopause and menopause with a good nutritional foundation is a powerful tool to protect our health from the natural changes that take place. We know, for instance, that stress gets our bodies primed to run away from lions (or deadlines) and ensures that more sugar stays in our blood for our muscles. When we do need to run away physically, the stress response is fantastic as you have more fuel to help make your escape. In our modern reality, however, that biscuit you nervously ate between meetings at your desk is simply keeping your blood sugar levels high for no reason.

So what should we eat, and how should we eat, to help mitigate the negative impacts that stress can have on our bodies? We can see that stress makes menopausal symptoms worse and finding ways of coping with stress is *hugely* helpful. Evidence shows that simple daily practices can have a great impact on mental wellbeing; breathwork for just 5 minutes every day can significantly reduce stress and anxiety levels. Breathing exercises can also be done anywhere at any time. Simply put a timer on your phone and spend 5 minutes breathing in and out, slowly and gently with your eyes closed or looking at a point like a favourite tree or a piece of art you love. I love lying down and popping on an eye mask with a simple breathing meditation to help me reset. There are countless books, apps, video tutorials and recorded meditations to help you find the breathwork that works for you, and it's something that is definitely worth trying.

When it comes to nourishment and stress, there are four main things I always keep in mind when I am trying to mitigate stress:

- **Remember to eat!** I often forget to have proper meals when I am under pressure and feeling stressed and will then eat a random much larger meal mid-afternoon when I realize I'm lacking nourishment. This leads to hunger, a lack of energy and results in a higher chance of suffering with more hormonal migraines.

- **Be mindful of sweet foods and milky chocolate.** The foods that we reach for at high times of stress can often make us feel more stressed. Research shows that cortisol impacts our sugar metabolism so we are more likely to crave sweet foods. Keep dark chocolate to hand but focus on vegetables and protein-rich foods first – like beans, mushrooms, eggs and leafy greens. For a super quick meal, just add some tinned fish, sustainably sourced where possible, to some rocket and add some mixed seeds and finish with a piece of fruit like an apple.

- **Think colourful.** Colourful foods contain more plant chemicals called polyphenols, which are nature's powerful antioxidants. These chemicals are there to protect plants against threats such as cold weather or pests and they actually help protect us against the negative impacts of stress. Berries, beetroot, dark leafy veg, cabbage, mushrooms, spices like turmeric, nuts and beans all contain plenty of polyphenols and will make your plate look very colourful.

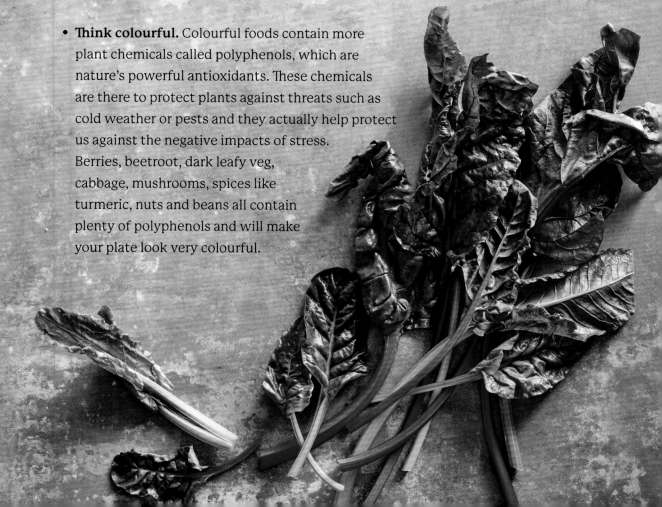

- **Enjoy eating.** It's easy to eat on the go, at our desks, on the phone or standing in the kitchen when we have a lot going on. Eating is one of life's simplest pleasures and enjoying our food is one of the best ways to make sure we are taking the opportunity to de-stress and focus on our food. This is also known as mindful eating, and it helps us to be more intuitive in how much we eat and what we choose to eat too. Sitting with family, friends or ourselves at a table with a plate of food we are paying attention to is an entirely different experience to mindlessly munching on something we've grabbed while reading an email or rushing to get to the next thing.

Movement — is movement medicine?

The science is clear that you can't out-train a bad diet. For healthy weight loss, exercise by itself does not work[24] and for most people, if you're looking for long-term sustainable weight loss, neither does dieting and restrictive calorie counting[25]. A lot of money has been spent on the science of exercise, and as mentioned earlier, food industry giants were very invested in making exercise the solution for our growing obesity epidemic instead of our food. What this has helped us do is understand two things: our food environment and access to healthy dietary choices are what is fuelling obesity, not a lack of exercise; and exercise is fundamental for health, but not in the way we might think.

I find that talking about exercise can be quite polarizing. Some of my clients are gym goers, some have personal trainers and some cringe at the idea of going to a gym. The thing is, exercise needn't be formal or structured, it doesn't require a membership or fancy machinery. A qualified, experienced personal trainer can be really helpful to start off with, to help you understand how to move and avoid injury. My clients are always surprised by the immediate impact just moving more in the day has on their health. You don't have to join the gym or book yourself into a yoga class, but what is definitely worth remembering is that movement is more than medicine, it is an essential part of life, whichever way you choose to do it.

Think through your usual day and make a note of when you might move and for how long. After waking up, many of us will have a fairly usual routine that may or may not involve walking the dog, dropping kids off at school, caring for grandkids or family members, or commuting to work. Some of us may do none of those things in the morning and automatically have one fewer movement opportunity built into the day. The majority of us will then spend prolonged periods of time in a fairly sedentary state. We might get up and go somewhere nearby to grab some lunch, or we might not. Some of us will eat our lunch and continue sitting

My clients are always surprised by the immediate impact just moving more in the day has on their health.

down until it's time to finish work or go home. Some of us might be able to fit in a visit to the gym, an exercise class, an at-home workout or another walk with the dog. This is so variable from person to person, and it really depends on where you are in your life at the moment. Some of my clients who are perimenopausal still have very young children and a career, so have very busy schedules, and some of my post-menopausal clients are no longer working and have found that the change in schedule has left them lacking opportunities to move. Many of my clients don't realize the pivotal role that movement plays in their metabolic and long-term health.

We know from the ZOE Menopause Study that after menopause, women are significantly worse at metabolizing glucose and they are also more likely to choose sugar-rich foods. When our bodies aren't effective at metabolizing glucose, it results in high blood-sugar concentrations for longer periods and insulin, which is normally very effective at moving blood sugar out of the blood and into our muscles, liver and fat tissues, becomes less effective. In the long term, this dysregulated sugar metabolism is more likely to cause type 2 diabetes, obesity, Alzheimer's[26] and liver disease, not to mention mood disorders, hunger and worse sleep. This is the main reason why so much dietary advice for menopausal and post-menopausal women focuses on reducing the amount of freely available sugar and refined carbohydrates in our diet.

So many of my menopausal clients say to me that they are eating exactly the same foods as they always have, but they feel dreadful and are gaining weight. The morning croissant, afternoon biscuits or sugar in your coffee have a completely different impact on your metabolism after menopause compared to when you were pre-menopausal. I think this is hard to accept, but equally powerful when embraced.

And why is this crucial in the context of movement? Because one of the simplest ways to help our bodies reduce high blood sugar levels when our metabolism is not as effective as it used to be, is to move our muscles. Our muscles prefer to use sugar for fuel, so one of the easiest things we can do to help regulate our blood sugar is to move after we eat. And by move, I mean a 20-minute walk, hoovering the house, dancing in your living room or anything else that involves moving your muscles. This is one of the simplest, most effective daily changes we can make for good health, but we have to factor it into our day and make it a priority so that it becomes second nature to get up and move after a meal.

> It turns out that we need to engage in resistance training activity at least twice per week to help maintain our muscle mass, as well as moving regularly every day.

A separate, equally important, point to make on the importance of movement is its role in muscle mass maintenance. Our skeletal muscles are what literally keep us standing, upright and strong enough to climb stairs and get up from chairs. This may seem simple enough now, but as we age the impact of muscle loss, which truly ramps up after the age of 45, is a major contributor to frailty, falls and metabolic disease. Maintaining muscle mass is a little bit more work than simply walking up the stairs or carrying our shopping bags in. It turns out that we need to engage in resistance training activity at least twice per week to help maintain our muscle mass, as well as moving regularly every day. Activities like dancing, lifting weights or doing some yoga all help with this.

Many of my clients have quite sedentary desk jobs that mean they rarely have the opportunity to walk or move around for very long. They will often tell me that they train at the gym two or three times per week, but these two types of movement are both necessary and one cannot compensate for the other. In other words, we ideally incorporate movement such as walking, taking the stairs and other exercise 'snacks' (see Lavina's section on movement) every day, plus we engage in some more structured strength training at least twice per week. This doesn't mean we will all become weightlifters, but it does mean that we can aim to engage in exercise which stimulates muscle growth and maintenance to make sure we are able to support our activity into older age.

The evidence on the benefits of exercise is staggering. While it is almost useless for any significant weight loss, it is instrumental in *maintaining* a healthy weight[27]. Much more than just weight, though, the impact of movement on mental health is well established, and there is some recent research, albeit a small study[28], which showed some really promising results. In this study, the physical intervention group simply received information on the benefits of movement and started with 30 minutes of movement every day (some stretching and walking for 20 minutes in week 1) to stretching and walking for 80 minutes by week 12. All menopausal symptoms, including heart palpitations, hot flushes, irritability, vaginal dryness and joint discomfort, significantly decreased in the activity group and did not improve at all for the control group. This is really encouraging and is something I have seen in my own clinic, with clients reporting that they feel an immediate benefit to their health when they make a daily lunchtime walk an integral part of their day.

The main thing to remember is that prioritizing movement as a key part of your day is a habit that needs to be set and reinforced *every* day. It is a non-negotiable part of maintaining our long-term health, as well as improving our symptoms, and becomes even more important for women after menopause. One of the hallmark metabolic changes seen in menopausal women is their worsened blood glucose response. This is a problem for many reasons, including increased risk of Alzheimer's and type 2 diabetes, and one of the most effective ways to reverse this risk in the long term is by maintaining good muscle mass and moving every day.

I am lucky to have Lavina Mehta MBE contribute her insight on menopause and exercise. She makes movement accessible for all and her own inspiring personal story and passion are infectious.

Movement and menopause
– Lavina Mehta MBE

I qualified as a personal trainer aged 40, after falling in love with what fitness and strength training did for my physical and mental health. I only started working out in my thirties and never really imagined it would become a new career, after leaving my job in the corporate world as a project manager in order to raise my three boys. After providing twice-daily workouts on my social media channels throughout the Covid pandemic, I was awarded an MBE for services to health and fitness in October 2020. My mission is to help all ages *Feel Good* physically and mentally, and to reduce the risks of common chronic diseases through Exercise Snacking, and my free *Feel Good* chair workouts. My slogan is to 'Exercise for Sanity not Vanity', as I am passionate about promoting the mental health benefits of exercise, which have got me through so many of life's challenges, especially the peri/menopause. I want everyone to focus less on how we look and more on how we feel! I am a proud Ambassador for Diabetes UK and the Alzheimer's Society and really want to break down the common barriers to exercise – time, cost and motivation – to get people moving for long-term health. Exercise and nutrition go hand-in-hand, especially in menopause – I believe in focusing on nurturing and nourishing your body, not depriving or restricting it.

I became a patron of the Menopause Mandate after sharing my own perimenopause journey on social media to help normalize the conversation, break the taboos, raise awareness, stop women from suffering in silence and help them feel empowered to find solutions. I struggled with my perimenopause since turning 40, but I truly believe the power of exercise and lifestyle changes can help women embrace this phase, like they have for me. Exercise is what has helped me stay strong, positive and manage my peri/menopausal symptoms, and thrive! Midlife is an opportunity for us all to invest in ourselves and focus on longevity and health.

Exercise to feel good in menopause

Exercise during menopause, especially strength training, is key for our bone, brain, heart, mental and long-term health. Women are more susceptible to chronic illnesses like heart disease, Alzheimer's, osteoporosis and diabetes during their midlife, but regular movement can help reduce these risks and future-proof you. By reframing our focus on health rather than just weight I want women to find joy in movement that builds confidence, consistency and sustainability.

I understand that working out can seem daunting or impossible when you're sleep deprived, lacking energy and motivation from experiencing peri/menopausal symptoms like hot flushes, joint pains, anxiety, low mood, disrupted sleep, and battling with the typical menopause weight gain, but exercise really can help to reduce them and, more often than not, these symptoms can be exacerbated by lack of movement. Exercise can provide a brilliant solution with or without HRT, alongside healthy eating and positive lifestyle changes. Exercise also helps manage symptoms by releasing feel-good endorphins that boost your mood and self-esteem. That's where my easy concept of Exercise Snacking comes in as the perfect solution to get started.

I want to help and empower women to navigate this journey holistically, with easy tools, especially during a challenging and demanding period, juggling families, work, elderly parents and children (in the 'sandwich' generation).

Let's get Exercise Snacking!

Rather than doing the typical 30/60 minutes of exercise all in one go, you can break it into smaller 'snacks', which have the same, if not greater, health benefits. Studies show that short bite-size chunks or bouts of movement throughout the day may be just as effective as doing it all at once. Remember that no amount is too small, even 2/5/10 minutes is beneficial.

I want to highlight that resistance/strength training is vital during this time, as our muscle mass declines after the age of 35 by approximately 3–5% a year. Building and preserving muscle mass is critical and the more lean muscle mass you have, the more insulin sensitivity and the more calories you'll burn, even at rest. We also need to keep our bones strong to reduce the risk of osteoporosis. During perimenopause itself, the loss of muscle and bone density increases. As oestrogen levels decline in menopause, this can lead to bone loss and low bone density. Once you are post-menopausal, this oestrogen loss accelerates and the decrease in muscle and bone mass is exacerbated further. Strength training is key to strengthening muscles, bones and joints; reducing body fat; building lean muscle; helping maintain a healthy weight, keeping our hearts and brains fit and subsequently reducing the risks of so many chronic illnesses. Lifting weights is a great antidepressant too, and keeps me sane. It's honestly my me-time, and makes me feel empowered, strong in both body and mind.

We want to build up gradually and snack our way to hitting the government guidelines of physical activity, which are 150 minutes of moderate intensity cardio or 75 minutes of vigorous cardio (or a combination of both) and strength training at least 2 times a week (but I'd prefer more!).

This can sound daunting, which is why breaking it up into small, quick, fun snacks is a great approach. Start off small (set yourself realistic snack-size goals), listen to your body and be kind to yourself. Finding movement you love is key to consistency and commitment, especially during menopause.

My ten top tips and snacks to get you started

1   Go for a 10-minute 'Feel Good Walk' outdoors (ideally in nature) after each meal or go for six 5-minute 'walk snacks' in the day.

2   Do a 2-minute 'HIIT Snack' when the kettle is boiling/veggies are steaming, like 30 seconds of star jumps, high knees, marching/ jogging on the spot and some boxing (add some bean cans as light weights). Add extra sets/longer rounds if you have more time.

3   Do a 5-minute 'Strength Snack' bodyweight workout while you're making your coffee/cooking (maybe a minute of squats, press-ups, dips, planks and lunges), then add weights as you progress.

4   Commit to a 'Squat Snack/Press-up Snack'– 3 sets of 10 reps – once a day, at your desk (home/office) or sofa even! Add some weights (cans/plastic bottles/rucksack or dumbbells) to progress.

5   Do a 'Balance Snack' – start with 10 seconds on each leg when you're brushing your teeth (build up to as long as possible).

6   Start 'Stair Snacking' – commit to three flights of stairs, three times a day, maybe before your meals (at work/home with your rucksack/ laundry/shopping bags).

7   Sitting too long? Set an alarm to do a 'Stretch or Mobility Desk Snack' every 2 hours (switch Zoom cameras off!).

8   Commit to a 2-minute 'Core Snack' when you wake up.

9   Treat yourself to a 'Stretch Snack' with some simple drills, morning or evening, focusing on your breath to alleviate stress, anxiety and aid muscle recovery.

10 Have a rest day to stretch, breathe, for selfcare, plan your next week (diarize your Exercise Snacks and workouts) and celebrate your wins in a journal.

Most importantly, enjoy your feel-good journey!

Find Lavina's Feel Good Workouts, Exercise Snacks and tips on all social media @feelgoodwithlavina and her website www.feelgoodwithlavina.com

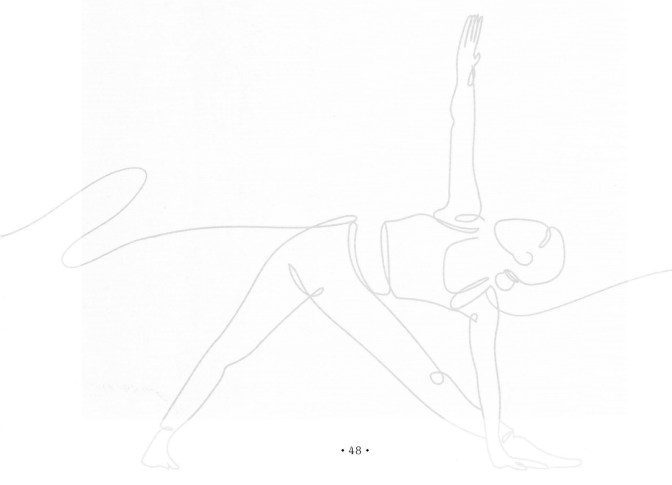

Mindfulness, enjoyment, and socializing: the pillars of social and spiritual wellbeing

Although I am a strong believer that nourishing food and daily movement are both essential components of a happy, long and healthy life, there is no denying that we are social creatures with a unique sense of self-awareness who thrive from their context. My own research looking at the importance of social function for better mental health opened my eyes to the power that community, access to trusted friends and family, freedom to work and ability to do things that we love have on our lives, even when other factors are quite bleak. The science behind the power of mindfulness and meditation is fascinating and absolutely convincing — it deserves a book of its own!

What's clear for women going through menopause and beyond is that having close trusted friendships, a support network and a degree of self-knowledge can make the world of difference to how we experience our everyday lives and how we feel about our future as a whole, which is very powerful.

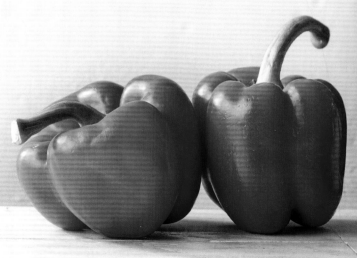

The Mediterranean Diet: the power of plants

The Mediterranean Diet (MeDi for short) is the most well researched, well understood, universally beneficial diet that we know of today. The data is so rich on this dietary pattern that we have the highest level of evidence available on its effects: systematic meta-reviews. These types of studies bring together data from hundreds of thousands of people across dozens of studies to understand the levels of impact on health outcomes. It's a comprehensive look at all of the evidence on a topic and can only be conducted when there are enough high-quality studies in well-conducted systematic reviews and meta-analyses to warrant combining them.

To put that into a research context, one well-conducted study is just one building block that will contribute to one systematic review (which may have 10–25 studies in it). A meta-review then collates around 10–30 of the systematic reviews and combines the data from them all to analyze the effect reported in the combined data from all of the studies. It's a complex piece of work, and one that really contributes to our level of confidence in the evidence. A famous randomized controlled trial which showed that following the Mediterranean Diet reduces severity of depression by 30% was inspired by previous reviews of the evidence[29]. One such super-review (or 636 studies) published in 2021 in the *European Journal of Public Health*[30] reported that following a Mediterranean Diet reduced the risk of dying of cancer by 14%, of cognitive decline and Alzheimer's by 40% and reduction in risk for death due to a heart attack by 68%. These results are astonishingly good. If the MeDi could be sold as a pill, we'd all be buying it! These are findings repeated across many studies in hundreds of thousands of people, so this is not a chance finding and it's something that we know has a positive impact.

Another benefit of the MeDi is that it is sustainable, focusing mostly on plant foods such as legumes, whole grains, seasonal fruits and vegetables, mushrooms, nuts and seeds and extra virgin olive oil, with moderate amounts of small oily fish, eggs, dairy and very occasional meat consumption. Unfortunately, our diets are moving away from this pattern as we all consume more pre-packaged and pre-prepared foods, meat and meat products daily, processed dairy products, pastries, confectionery, muffins and pizzas instead of the whole foods which feature in the MeDi. Some recent evidence suggests that following a MeDi pattern could not only decrease our risk of chronic diseases after menopause, which we know are increased in post-menopausal women, but also improve the symptoms of menopause[31]. A 2013 cohort study of over 6,000 women showed that following a Mediterranean Diet reduced the risk of vasomotor menopausal symptoms (hot flushes, night sweats) by about 20%[32], which is a reduction in risk which all of my clients and friends who suffer with these symptoms would gladly take.

The menopause science that changed my life

The most recent evidence on the impact that diet can have on menopausal symptoms comes from colleagues at ZOE. Two studies from the smartphone-based ZOE Health Study investigated how weight and diet quality impact menopausal symptoms. In a peer-reviewed abstract accepted for the prestigious IUNS conference, the ZOE Health Profile study of over 25,000 women found that body weight (measured as BMI) had a significant impact on the likelihood of suffering with menopausal symptoms. Mood changes were found in nearly 60% of women with a healthy weight, but in nearly 70% of women suffering with severe obesity, with a significant difference also observed in likelihood of hot flushes between women of a healthy weight (54%) and those with severe obesity (66%).

The ZOE PREDICT-1 Menopause study published in *The Lancet*[33] was an in-depth analysis to understand how many menopausal symptoms are due to hormone changes as opposed to biological ageing. An interview I did with British newspaper *The Times* to report this new research is what led me to write, speak and eventually write this book on the topic of nutrition and menopause – because the potential to improve millions of women's experience of menopause and beyond is hugely exciting.

Data on diet, heart and metabolic health, gut microbiome, blood sugar and blood fat response to a standardized meal were all recorded in post-menopausal women and women of the same age who had not yet gone through menopause, as well as a group of age-matched men. These comparisons showed a clear difference in post-menopausal women – who had poorer blood sugar response, decreased sleep quality and a tendency to eat more sugary foods when compared to the women of the same age who were pre-menopausal. Some of the unfavourable effects of menopause on health were found to be mediated in part by diet and the gut microbiome, which also showed several changes post-menopause. The results show that a powerful shift occurs in a woman's metabolism and gut microbiome composition, affecting her gut health and metabolism during perimenopause and after menopause. This study is a fundamental piece of research which helps to explain the mechanisms by which so many of the menopausal changes experienced by women actually take place.

Key findings in menopausal women:

- Increased inflammation and blood sugar responses after eating.

- Negative effects on blood sugar control (a key risk factor of cardiovascular disease and type 2 diabetes), showing for the first time this is not just an inevitable part of ageing.

- Higher body fat percentage and increased inflammation.

- Post-menopausal women are more likely to consume more dietary sugars and report poorer sleep compared with women of the same age.

- The impact of being overweight or having obesity on the increased likelihood of suffering from the main symptoms of menopause.

- Increased presence of pro-inflammatory and obesogenic microbiome strains.

In order to understand the impact of menopause on metabolic health changes, ZOE PREDICT investigated the changes in metabolic responses in pre- peri- and post-menopausal women. Fasting blood glucose levels, inflammation and sugar intakes were all higher in post-menopausal women. Moreover, blood glucose, fat and insulin levels were all higher post-menopause, contributing to a higher likelihood of type 2 diabetes, cardiovascular disease and obesity, already associated with oestrogen decline in post-menopausal women.

THE GOOD NEWS

Unpublished, newly analyzed data provides evidence to show that diet – not only what but how we eat – can transform a woman's menopausal symptoms. Women who were overweight or suffered from obesity were much more likely to report symptoms, including anxiety, joint pain, low libido and weight gain. Following a healthy plant-based diet was shown to be protective against symptoms, with women who consumed the most whole plants in their diet much less likely to suffer from any symptoms, even if they were already overweight. Hot flushes and sleep disturbances, which are considered the most debilitating symptoms by many women, were 30% less likely to be reported by women who ate plenty of healthy whole plant foods in their diet, irrespective of their weight. This is huge, brilliant news for women everywhere because we can improve our quality of life right now and for the future by adding more plants to our plates.

This evidence shows that while it's important to keep a healthy body weight throughout life and through menopause, eating a healthy plant-based diet is much more important than restrictive dieting. Adding plants to your plate will likely help with menopause symptoms, regardless of weight and HRT use. It is the first time that this kind of research has been done in such a large group of perimenopausal women and it offers further insight into how we can support our health through this change.

By incorporating new scientific learnings about menopause into the diet, women can reduce the unfavourable health impacts associated with menopause, either directly by reducing inflammation and blood sugar spikes or indirectly by altering the gut microbiome. Simple changes include increasing consumption of whole plants, reducing ultra-processed carbohydrates and incorporating more high-fibre and high-polyphenol foods every day.

When we take a look at the evidence overall, there is a strong argument for adopting the MeDi as a woman preparing for or going through menopause, or adjusting to life post-menopause. It is possible to decrease the likelihood of cognitive decline, depression, cancer, hot flushes and heart disease, simply by changing your food to follow this pattern. Here are some simple swaps and foods to add to your plate that can help make that change without too much effort:

- Rice ▷ pearled barley
- White pasta ▷ spelt pasta
- Couscous ▷ buckwheat
- Iceberg lettuce ▷ colourful lollo rosso or rocket
- Minced meat bolognese ▷ black beans and mushroom bolognese
- White sandwich loaf bread ▷ seeded rye sourdough bread
- Canned tuna ▷ canned mackerel
- Breakfast cereal or muesli ▷ overnight oats with kefir and nuts (see page 92)
- Flavoured low-fat dessert ▷ seasonal fruit salad (see page 196)
- Milk chocolate ▷ dark chocolate (70% cocoa solids or more)
- Sweet pastries or pancakes ▷ protein pancakes with blueberries
- Store-bought salad vinaigrette ▷ homemade extra virgin olive oil and apple cider vinegar dressing
- A handful of spinach, kale or cabbage added to soups or steamed as a side

The MeDi could save millions in healthcare costs by reducing disease burden and disability, and it is helpful for the planet too. Creating a food environment where choosing whole grains and fresh vegetables is as easy and convenient as picking up a ready meal or a takeaway is something that requires a concerted effort from our governments as well as ourselves.

With this book, I hope to arm you with the knowledge you need to make daily choices to improve your future health and positively influence the health of those important to you. It's a well-known fact that it is still the women in society who choose, prepare and provide most of the food for their families. Jane's delicious recipes hold the MeDi spirit at their heart, and they all have the key principles of the MeDi for health.

Nightcaps and midnight snacks: creating healthy habits

Alcohol and menopause

There are many reasons why it is worth watching our alcohol intake. At a basic level, alcohol is a carcinogenic neurotoxin, meaning it can cause cancer and is toxic to the cells of our nervous system, including our brains. I think it's worth remembering this fundamental detail when talking about alcohol, because the fact that it is a socially acceptable drug doesn't make it any less dangerous. In certain cultures, it can even feel socially essential — 'going for a drink' is as pervasive as 'grabbing a bite to eat' in countries around the world. Social interaction is very important for health but the consequences of drinking in excess are staggeringly negative. In a startling analysis by Professor David Nutt and his team, the harm to society and to self which drinking alcohol causes in comparison to other drugs is pretty sobering[34].

Unfortunately, alcohol negatively impacts women's health harder and faster than men. The negative impacts in women include higher risk of inflammation in the brain, alcohol-related heart disease and immune diseases and the now very-well-established risk of alcohol consumption and oestrogen-sensitive breast cancer[35]. Some studies report an increased risk of breast cancer as high as an extra 12% per drink per day. This is explained by alcohol's interaction with oestrogen-specific receptors, changing their structure and function. Alcohol also damages a woman's liver more severely than it does a man's liver, at lower levels of consumption and over a shorter period of time.

Reading that paragraph might cause you to consider going teetotal, or you may already have given up drinking or you may be one of the rare (but growing) number of women who have never drunk alcohol. Drinking alcohol is highly personal, and its effects will vary widely between individuals. The key is to understand the risks, recognize when alcohol is becoming a temporary solution for a long-term problem and ask for help if you need it. For everyone reading this who wants to enjoy an occasional drink, the science is simple.

The 'French Paradox' is the term given to the epidemiological finding that French people generally suffer with less heart disease, despite their love of butter and cheese. Scientists have investigated whether their daily glass of red wine is to thank for this, and there is evidence to support the idea that a small amount of red wine spread over a week (one unit per day, which is less than one small glass, so for pragmatic reasons I like to think of this as three glasses on three separate evenings of the week) can be beneficial. There's also some good science to explain what is so special about red wine and why it might actually reduce inflammation[36]. The key here is to remember that dose is so important. Any beneficial effects of the many chemical compounds found in red wine are nullified if too much is consumed, as alcohol is still problematic.

There is virtually no evidence to support other types of alcohol drinking, and even for red wine drinking it is very much within a Mediterranean Diet pattern of drinking a glass of red with your meal, with friends. Personally, I recommend that my clients who have a healthy relationship with alcohol continue to drink a glass of red wine with a meal no more than three nights per week. For women who are menopausal later than 51 or have other factors that increase their risk of oestrogen-sensitive breast cancer, I recommend that they don't drink regularly at all.

IS SUGAR TO BLAME?

Blood sugar levels, also known as blood glucose levels, peaks, rollercoasters and glycaemic response, have received a lot of attention as a marker of wellbeing in the past five years or so. I think this is partly because people have become more aware of the important impact sugar has on our health and partly because continuous glucose monitors (CGMs) have become more mainstream, and low sugar diets (low carb) have become popular too. When COVID-19 struck and people with type 2 diabetes (T2D) were more than twice as likely to become severely ill and to die[37], more people became interested in proactively reducing their risk of diabetes or trying to reverse their diabetes with diet.

I have no doubt that a better understanding of our bodies' ability to effectively control blood sugar levels is hugely helpful in improving our health, slowing the ageing process, reducing the risk of T2D and obesity, as well as improving energy levels throughout the day. The work that my colleagues at ZOE do both with the ZOE PREDICT studies[38] and ongoing studies powered by our users have shown how different we all are in our responses to blood sugar, and what these different responses might mean for our health, sleep, mood and hunger. When I did my own ZOE test, I realized that my blood sugar control isn't as smooth and seamless as I'd hoped, which makes sense as there is a family history of diabetes. Type 2 diabetes does have a strong genetic component, which goes some way in explaining why South Asians, for example, are four times more likely to develop the disease[39]. There are other factors which increase risk, like having obesity, gestational diabetes in pregnancy and weight gain (from 5kg/11lb upward sees the steepest increase in risk). So what actually causes weight gain and a genetic predisposition to lead to T2D? Let's start from the beginning.

Glucose metabolism

This is going to get a bit scientific, but I think it's really worth understanding. Carbohydrates are a complex group of chemicals present in our food. When thinking about carbohydrates that have an impact on our blood glucose, we are talking about glycaemic carbohydrates that cause a change in blood glucose levels. Non-glycaemic carbohydrates have no impact on our blood glucose, as we cannot absorb them, and they include things like cellulose (from plant cell walls) and inulin (the fibre in chicory root). Glucose is a form of carbohydrate, which is our bodies' preferred form of energy. It is a type of monosaccharide because it travels in a unit of one (mono). Sucrose (table sugar), lactose (the sugar in milk) and other disaccharides are, you guessed it, made of two units of carbohydrates linked together. At a cellular level, glucose is the final substance that enters our tissues and

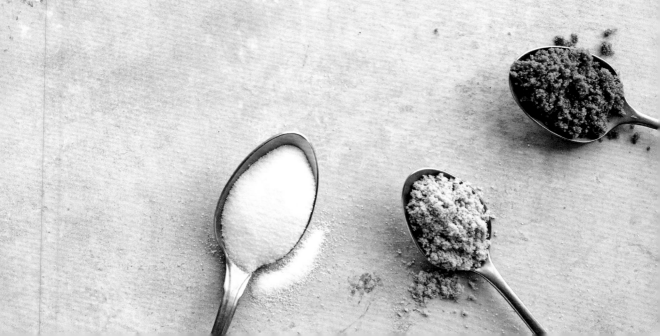

converts to ATP, which is the energy currency of our entire bodies, needed for everything from muscle contraction and neurotransmitter signalling, to making new cells.

Specific enzymes in our saliva, and some released by our pancreas, break larger starches down into glucose, which is then absorbed through the cell membrane and into our cells in the small intestine. These broken-down sugars travel via the portal vein to the liver, which is the organ that uses the glucose for metabolic reactions. The liver is an amazing organ which requires a lot of energy as it is responsible for thousands of processes, including making new proteins and creating glucose from chemicals called ketones when we have long periods of fasting. It is impossible to have good blood sugar control without a healthy liver.

After we eat, any sugar left over from these metabolic reactions in the liver ends up in our blood, and when our pancreatic cells sense a rise in sugar levels, they release the hormone insulin, which works hard to clear the glucose out of our blood. One of the ways it does this is to tell our liver to store some glucose as glycogen, which it then re-releases into the blood once blood sugar levels start to fall, to keep blood sugar dips, peaks and rollercoasters to a minimum. Glycogen is also the storage unit for glucose in our muscles and is released back into the blood as glucose when needed. This is because when our blood glucose levels fall too low, we can go into hypoglycaemia (low blood sugar), which can leave us feeling hungry, shaky, faint and can be very dangerous for prolonged periods, sometimes resulting in loss of consciousness and even coma.

When our blood sugar level is low and we need more energy, glucagon is the hormone that is released. Glucagon has the exact opposite effect to insulin: it releases glucose from cells back into the blood to increase blood sugar levels. This insulin and glucagon balancing act is important for our organs, tissues and cells. Aside from the liver, muscle, kidney and cells of the gut lining, when glucose is taken up into cells, it cannot be re-released into our blood. It can only be stored and used for the energy currency (ATP) just mentioned. This is really important to remember because flooding our cells with glucose at a higher rate than our cells can use the energy for ATP is a main driver for ageing and disease. It's a bit like adding far too much fuel to a running engine: it eventually floods and either blows up or stops working altogether.

The liver and muscle cells that can store and release glycogen have a limit on how much they can store. Having more muscle means we have more glycogen storage space, and we have more muscles to use that store, which is why strength training and maintaining good muscle mass is so helpful for good metabolic health (see Lavina's box on page 44). Our liver can become bigger (or enlarged) as it tries to accommodate more storage, but this is not a good thing and results in inflammation and even non-alcoholic fatty liver disease (NAFLD). When the storage space for glycogen is 'full', the

It's really worth noting that stress is intrinsically linked with our metabolic health — you cannot eat yourself healthy in a state of chronic stress.

liver moves to transforming the excess glucose into fatty acids, more specifically very low density lipoproteins (v-LDL, the very bad type of cholesterol) to be transported throughout blood vessels to fat tissues for storage. This goes some way to explaining why eating lots of avocados and walnuts, naturally high in fats, is much less likely to cause your bad cholesterol to go up, whereas eating lots of pastries, sugary drinks and highly processed biscuits is very likely to.

The good news is that a simple overnight fast releases enough glucagon to stimulate glycogen release from the liver, freeing up room in the 'storage unit', which is one of the reasons why giving yourself a good 12–14 hours without food overnight between dinner and breakfast is a good idea.

To add to this already complex picture, stress hormones like cortisol also impact blood sugar levels, making sure we have enough blood sugar to 'fight or flight'. Our pancreas is also connected to our nervous system, and sends signals to our brain if our blood sugar levels are changing erratically and causing a stress response. As you can imagine, this means that being chronically stressed and eating foods that cause rapid and continuous changes to our blood sugar levels can cause high blood glucose levels and a higher risk of developing type 2 diabetes[40]. Stress has a huge impact on all of the body. In fact, stress and its cousin, inflammation, are the two necessary physiological responses that cause the most damage when they are repeatedly activated outside of their original purpose. It's really worth noting that stress is intrinsically linked with our metabolic health — you cannot eat yourself healthy in a state of chronic stress.

WHAT'S FAT AND WEIGHT GAIN GOT TO DO WITH IT?

Hopefully now you have a good overview of how our body absorbs, breaks down, uses, stores and regulates our favourite energy source. So what happens when our diet pushes these pathways off balance? And how does menopause make women more susceptible to this shift in increased fat mass?

One of the most hated 'side effects' of menopause is the increased fat around the waist that women suddenly develop during perimenopause, often called the 'menopause belly'. This added fat deposit is actually a result of hormonal changes, as well as metabolic changes, as our bodies desperately try to make up for the falling levels of oestrogen to achieve homeostasis. This is because fat is an effective hormone tissue in its own right and it can release oestrogen into the blood, so our bodies helpfully accumulate extra fat to make extra oestrogen when they sense that circulating oestrogen is falling. This simple solution does not solve the falling oestrogen levels (but does go some way to explaining why women with obesity have higher circulating oestrogen levels and a later average age of menopause), and the accumulation of fatty tissue is made worse by poorer glucose metabolism caused by menopause.

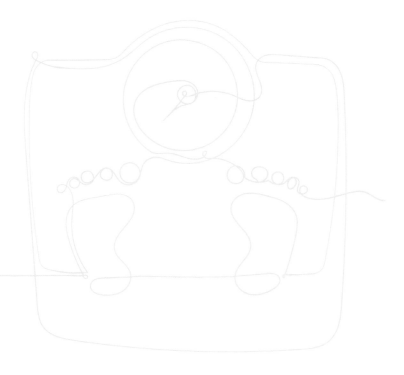

The Diet & Menopause ZOE study explored the impact of dietary quality and health status in around 10,000 perimenopausal women. The most commonly reported symptoms included sleep problems (81–84% of women), anxiety (65–72%), mood changes (57–70%) and hot flushes (62–69%). Women who were overweight or had obesity were much more likely to experience menopausal symptoms including chills, thinning of hair or dry skin, hot flushes, mood changes and sleep problems.

The most commonly reported menopausal symptoms included sleep problems (81–84% of women), anxiety (65–72% of women), mood changes (57–70%) and hot flushes (62–69%).

We've talked about the fact that our liver and muscles have a finite storage capacity for glycogen (the storage format of glucose). We've also seen how the liver turns to making sugars into fats when that glycogen store is full up (or in the case of fructose, which can't be stored as glycogen and so goes straight to fatty acid synthesis). Those fats then travel in our blood to be taken into fat stores as long-term energy storage but may get stuck in blood vessels along the way and contribute to plaques, which clog up our blood vessels and cause inflammation because they are very 'sticky'.

So far, so good. Insulin drives extra glucose into our liver, muscles and fat cells after we have eaten and have higher blood glucose, while glucagon kicks into action to help release energy when it's needed – because we haven't eaten for a while or have done a lot of movement – from liver and muscle glycogen stores, as well as from fat cells.

In the simplest of terms, weight gain of fat tissue happens when we have lots of opportunities for insulin to store energy for later, and not enough opportunities for glucagon to help release some of this energy back from storage. Insulin and glucagon cannot happen together, which is why hyperinsulinemia (high insulin levels throughout the day) is one of the signs of metabolic disease. This is not to do with exercise and definitely not to do with 'calories in, calories out'; this is about our 24-hour day and having time to cycle from 'eating and storing' to 'fasting and using' throughout the day. The more we signal our bodies to 'store energy', the more energy we store as fat in our fatty tissues, which in turn causes us to gain weight.

Basal metabolic rate (BMR) is a measure of how much energy our bodies need just to keep us alive without taking into account any movement or other increase in energy needs. It's what your body uses when you are lying still but awake, doing nothing else. If we have more muscle mass, this rate is higher. This basal rate decreases with age, so our body needs less energy to keep us alive as we age, meaning that by age 75, we need less fuel to stay alive than we did at 25. Going back to our engine analogy and thinking about glucose as the fuel we need, that fuel requirement goes down as we get older, and our cells (engines) will get more easily flooded or blown up too.

Our fat cells also have a 'limit' to how much fat they can store before becoming too full. They then start sending out distress signals to the rest of the body to say there is a malfunction. This fatty tissue malfunction is one of the biggest causes of excess inflammation in the bodies of people who are overweight and have obesity. Oestrogen is protective against this kind of fat tissue inflammation; in fact oestrogen receptors are found throughout fat tissue because the two are so intrinsically linked. Oestrogen can encourage the fat cells to release fatty acids like turning on a tap[41], and in animal models we can actually see that removing local oestrogen production causes obesity and insulin resistance. So yes, menopause can literally make us fat, and not because we have changed the way we eat; but because what we eat can change the course of this metabolic switch.

There's some fascinating research on fatty tissue and how it behaves essentially as a separate organ with its own hormones and regulatory processes. Our fat organ communicates with the rest of our body and does its best to regulate our stores to remain constant. In pre-menopausal women, much of this fat store is under the skin, in the bum and thighs, conferring a pear-shape. Post-menopause, women are much more likely to have an apple-shaped fat distribution, which is caused by fat accumulation around the organs in our abdomen and is associated with heart disease. Our oestrogen levels pre-menopause actually protect us from this more inflammatory type of fat storage, so we have to be more mindful of excess fat stores post-menopause.

We are surrounded by foods with freely available instant energy starches everywhere we go, so it's easy to see how we have gradually slipped into daily habits of lots of eating and storing, and not enough fasting and releasing. Food adverts reach us hundreds of times every day through social media, advertising and other media encouraging us to have a snack, grab a bite or enjoy an energy-boosting drink. The industry is doing what

Store
energy
as fat

Fasted

Stable
sugar
levels

Eating

Release
stored
energy

it needs to do to make more money and that means making us consume more of the product: food. What's really crucial to note here, and as many of us know, is that you don't need to be eating lots of food for this to happen. Eating starchy foods (think rice cakes, dates, a biscuit, a cracker etc) little and often for most of the day will also encourage our bodies to store weight as fat because the mechanisms remain the same.

If you give people food with added sugar, they eat a lot more of that food than they would without the added sugar, regardless of its overall macronutrient content.

After consistently high blood sugar levels over many years, our bodies start getting a bit tired and don't respond so well: this is called insulin resistance. What's known as insulin sensitivity simply refers to how well our tissues do the job of moving blood sugar out of the blood and into our cells. A hallmark sign of type 2 diabetes is insulin insensitivity (resistance), whereby your tissues basically stop responding properly to insulin and don't bring your blood sugar levels down properly. Once tissues have become insulin insensitive, our pancreas has to work harder to make more insulin in the hope of a response from the tissues. Insulin is also driving fatty acids into our fat tissues to make them store more fat. This is a simplified pathway to type 2 diabetes and fat weight gain. Luckily for us, our bodies are so adaptive that in the majority of cases it is reversible with diet and lifestyle changes alone.

So is sugar to blame? Yes and no. As we've covered earlier, all foods are converted to glucose for energy at a cellular level because it is necessary for our energy currency, ATP, to function. So fearing glucose is like fearing oxygen: it's pretty nonsensical. What is problematic is having so much glucose readily available in its simple forms (i.e. added sugars, refined starches and sugar in drinks) that our body absorbs and then has to try and store way more than it actually needs. Drawing on the oxygen comparison again, there is such a thing as oxygen toxicity too, so you can always have too much of a good thing.

The problem is that the more added sugar a food contains, the more we eat. That's right — if you give people food with added sugar, they eat a lot more of that food than they would without the added sugar, regardless of its overall macronutrient content. We just love the taste of free sugar, and our biology tells us to eat more of that food. This has served our ancestors and even some modern hunter gatherers well, who get as much as 70% of their energy requirement from honey or sweet berries when they become available to them. The difference is, of course, that they don't eat these foods every day, and often these foods will form the majority of energy intake at specific time points when other food is scarce. On top of that, a sugary meal is also likely to result in feeling hungrier later in the day when your blood sugar levels drop thanks to all the insulin your pancreas has pumped out, and your body signals you to find some more sugar to make sure you don't go into low sugar level territory (hypoglycaemia). So the devil is in the dose and, with sugar, the higher the dose in your food, the worse off you're likely to be in terms of blood sugar control, hunger and healthy weight maintenance.

What is the right dose?

Let's take a chickpea as an example of the importance of our food choices. Starches found in whole foods like chickpeas need to be broken down into simple sugars. Chewing the chickpea breaks down some of the plant cells and releases some starch which will either be broken down and absorbed, or released to provide food for our gut microbes (more on that later). Similarly, the fats found in chickpeas need to be 'released' from the cell and then broken down and absorbed by chewing and digesting the whole chickpea.

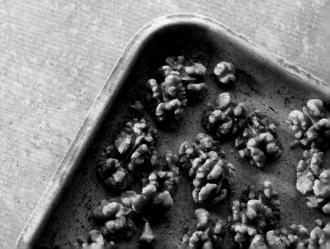

Let's look now at a popular 'chickpea puff' snack. Technically, the snack is made of chickpeas so it has the same starches, the same amount of fat and should have the same impact on our bodies if we are to believe that food labels tell us all we need to know about food. This chickpea puff, however, has been processed to make the chickpeas into a fine powder, which can

> Eating food in its original form is one of the easiest ways we can help improve our bodies' response to that food. It's as simple as that!

then be reconstituted into a crunchy snack shape not at all resembling a chickpea, and destroying the structure which made the fats and sugars more difficult to access in the process. So now we have very easy-to-absorb fats and sugars packaged and advertised as a healthy snack from a food that in its original form is delicious and healthy. This is the first problem with ultra-processed foods (UPFs). A randomized crossover trial (gold standard human study) on the difference between eating whole almonds and ground almonds showed that there was a significant change in how much fat was absorbed, depending on whether the almonds were whole or ground[42].

Eating food in its original form is one of the easiest ways we can help improve our bodies' response to that food. It's as simple as that! Making our bodies work for the nutrients by having to actually chew whole food is a great way of reducing the excess absorption of sugar and fat that is made available to us through ultra-processed ready-to-eat foods. The second part of the puzzle is about timing. As mentioned earlier, our bodies are tuned to go through periods of feeding and periods of fasting, but modern Western diets have completely changed that. It's not unusual to wake up and have a tea or coffee with milk and sugar within half an hour and to have our last food or drink, like a hot chocolate or a piece of fruit, half an hour before going to bed. If we are awake for at least 14 hours, from 8am to 10pm for example, this leaves only 10 hours overnight for our body to have a rest from metabolizing food, assuming we don't then also wake in the night looking for a snack. What's more, being tired and losing sleep causes us to crave more sugary foods, and having more glucose and insulin spikes that result from the sugary foods throughout the day are more likely to cause restless sleep and feeling less alert the next day[43]. Just breaking that cycle with a good overnight fast and reducing ultra-processed packaged foods can help restore energy levels and create more time for our bodies to repair and rebalance.

Sleep and menopause

One of the most common symptoms of menopause is night sweats and sleep disturbances. It may be the first symptom a woman notices which prompts her to ask for help, since not getting a good night's sleep is so disruptive to life in general. In the ZOE Menopause study[44], 12% of menopausal women had problems sleeping and 12% had higher sugar intake, significantly higher than pre-menopausal women. There are some key steps we can take to help our bodies effectively regulate our blood sugar levels and also improve our sleep quality:

- **Focus on whole foods first at every meal:** leafy greens, fresh herbs, eggs, nuts, vegetables (cooked or raw), whole grains, beans (fresh, canned or dried and soaked), pulses, seeds, fresh whole fruit with the skin on, fish, meat and fermented dairy products like kefir and natural yogurt.

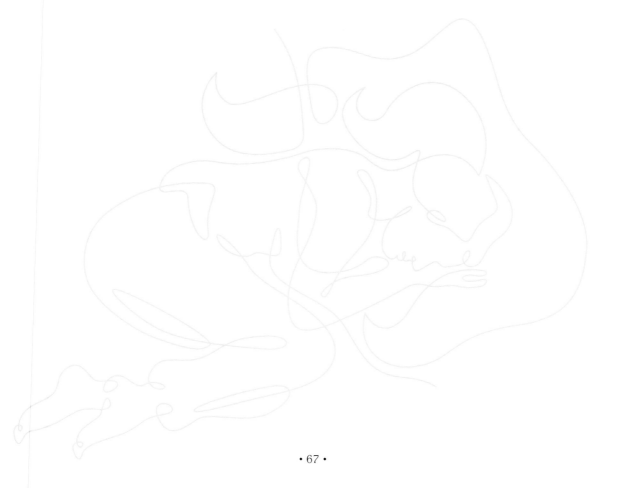

- **Try to have the same 10-hour eating window every day,** leaving a 12—14 hour overnight fast. For example, if you have breakfast at 8am every morning, try to have dinner by 6pm. Consistency is more important than perfection; there will be days when this is not possible!

- **Reduce refined carbohydrate and ultra-processed food consumption to occasional days.** Remove biscuits, pastries, doughnuts, chocolate bars, sweetened and low-fat yogurt, ready-made desserts, cakes and pre-packaged snack bars from your weekly shop.

- **Help your body keep blood glucose levels in check, by doing 10—20 minutes of brisk movement after meals.** Muscles moving primarily use glucose, making this the simplest way to reduce blood glucose levels and movement throughout the day is associated with better sleep, energy levels the next day and a myriad of benefits for our mood and healthier ageing.

Getting a good night's rest is absolutely essential, not only for our metabolic health as I've described above, but also for our brains. The brain has its own lymphatic system, known as the glymphatic system, which is a network of waste disposal for our brain cell channels, which only activates when we sleep. Knowing this, it is not surprising then that chronic lack of sleep is associated with brain diseases such as Alzheimer's. Another organ that benefits from an overnight fast and a rest from breaking down and absorbing food is our gut, and more specifically the trillions of microbes that live inside it.

The mighty microbiome

Our gut is phenomenally long, at least 4.5 metres (15ft), with 2.8–4.8 metres (9–16ft) of small intestine and about 1.5 metres (5ft) of large intestine. I remember during one of my work shadowing placements I attended surgery with a gastroenterology (gut) surgeon who let me observe as he worked. I was fascinated by just how much could fit in one person's body! For a long time the gut was overlooked, but we now know it is integral to our immune system function. The gut is amazing as an organ to witness with the naked eye, and that is nothing compared to what is going on at a microscopic level.

The entire length of our gut — from small intestine to the rectum — is a single cell layer of tiny fingers that stick into the middle of the gut (see diagram overleaf). These tiny fingers are called villi, and they continuously come into contact with our food as it passes through the long tube that is our gut, absorbing sugars, fats, proteins, water and nutrients at the top, and leaving more water and fibre to be passed further along to the large bowel. The chemistry that happens in the small intestine is absolutely crucial for good nutrient absorption and it's made possible by a healthy pancreas and liver, but also by the microbes that live in and colonize the villi.

The populations of microbes that live in our gut change as you travel down from the small intestine to the large intestine, with fewer species able to survive the alkaline pH in the small intestine, due to high concentrations of bile, and quite fast transit time of food through this part of the gut. As you travel further down the gut to the large intestine (aka colon), the pH changes to slightly acidic and the remaining food moves through a lot more slowly, leading to the most diverse community of microbes thriving here. There are more microbial cells in the human body than there are human cells, which means we are actually more bug than human. Technically, the correct term for us is a 'superorganism' — a communal group of human and microbial cells working together to stay alive and thrive.

These gut microbes have become quite famous in the past decade or so. Where we used to think that all bacteria were something to get rid of ASAP with antibiotics, we now know that these tiny organisms actually keep us alive. We know from mouse models and some very rare human examples that having no microbes in the gut leads to a fatal lack of

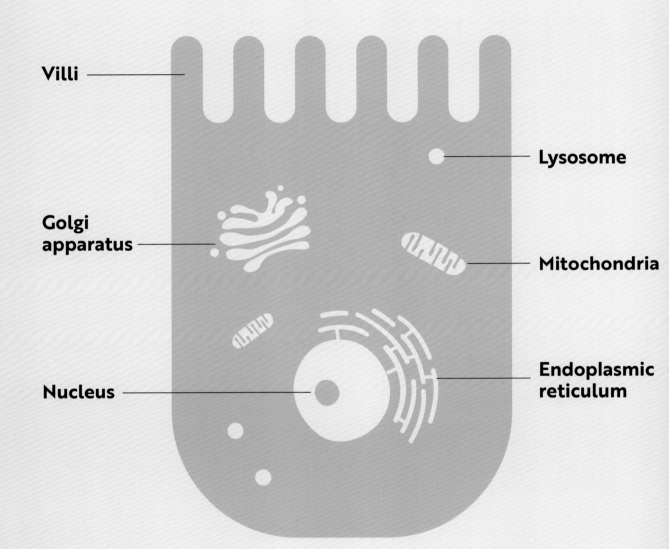

Villi

Golgi
apparatus

Nucleus

Lysosome

Mitochondria

Endoplasmic
reticulum

immune system function and eventually death. In fact, we evolved to live symbiotically with our microbes, so it's impossible for us to thrive without them. As we saw earlier, we even know that our gut microbes directly impact our mental health, and there are many other things they do, from impacting our likelihood of allergies to impacting the outcome of chemotherapy treatment[45].

To borrow Professor Tim Spector's analogy: the gut microbiome is like a garden which we need to tend to make sure it thrives. Think of the soil as the prebiotic fibres which arrive in the gut. They provide the nutrients and the anchor for the gut microbes. The gut microbes are the flowers, plants and grasses that grow in that soil and make a beautiful flourishing garden; the more diverse types of plants present, the richer the garden. A garden needs water, sunlight and occasionally some new seeds added to it; think of these as plant chemicals called polyphenols, fibre from fibre-rich foods and probiotic foods providing some new microbes to the mix. If we follow this analogy, a healthy thriving gut garden will produce beautiful flowers, plenty of oxygen, and will help preserve the health of the soil it lives in too. The postbiotic chemicals (also known as metabolites) that our gut microbes produce are like the flowers and oxygen of the gut garden that we directly benefit from.

So what is the opposite of a healthy, flourishing garden? A barren, dry land with no diversity and a soil that is unable to provide nutrients for growth. An arid landscape that is impacted by a lack of diversity, unhelpful chemicals disrupting plant growth, cracked earth and perhaps some weeds, but very little in the way of flowers. This is the garden equivalent of a gut that has very little fibre, suffers with constipation, is often exposed to chemicals or drugs that reduce the likelihood of helpful microbe colonization and may result in irritable bowel syndrome. This gut garden can't protect its soil and there is more likely to be damage to the barrier with lots of unwanted weeds and water lost from the soil.

CAN THE GUT MICROBIOME BE A POWERFUL TOOL THROUGH MENOPAUSE?

Good gut health is important throughout our lives, but it is especially helpful in protecting women's wellbeing during and after menopause. Menopause is marked by a range of hormonal changes which are known to impact gut health, causing symptoms such as irritable bowel, as well as changes in appetite regulation, heart health, cognition and metabolism. The close link between gut microbiome diversity and hormone regulation has led to research focusing on what is known as the estrobolome. The estrobolome is the microbial control centre in our gut that regulates the oestrogen available in our bodies. A healthy estrobolome is able to metabolize inactive oestrogens and phytoestrogens back to available circulating oestrogens, which can then act on oestrogen receptors all over the body, reducing the symptoms associated with menopause but also with a range of diseases.

After menopause, women are at a higher risk of obesity, certain types of cancer, cardiovascular disease and decreased cognitive function, all of which are associated with an increase in inflammation and changes in the diversity of our gut microbiome. Changing our diet to support gut microbiome diversity effectively improves markers of inflammation and improves oestrogen circulation, making it a promising and exciting new approach to improving post-menopausal women's wellbeing.

THE ESTROBOLOME – THE BODY'S SECRET HORMONE CONTROL CENTRE

The estrobolome is like a specialist team of gut bugs. These bugs make enzymes that help detach oestrogen from its receptors and break it back down into an active form. If your diet does not support a diverse gut microbiome, it can become imbalanced with fewer helpful gut microbes and less diversity. If the estrabolome is not working well for you, it could lead to lower levels of circulating oestrogen in your body. Supporting the estrabolome could help reduce menopausal symptoms in perimenopausal women, however it may also contribute to too much circulating oestrogen in post-menopausal women, which can have a negative impact. The science in this field is rapidly evolving and could hold the keys to some exciting treatments or screening tools in the future[46]. A recent study found that after menopause, women's gut bacteria become more like men of the same age than those of pre-menopausal women[47]. This changed microbiome is linked to lower levels of oestrogen and progesterone, a hallmark of the menopause transition. The study suggests that menopause depletes specific gut bacteria that are involved in hormone-related metabolic processes. There is also evidence to suggest that certain gut bacteria could reactivate sex hormones in post-menopausal women. Menopause-related gut microbiome changes are also linked with worse heart and metabolic disease risk in post-menopausal women, showing once again the important role that gut bacteria play in women's health during and after menopause.

We've seen that an early reduction in circulating oestrogens before the age of 50 may contribute to the development of conditions including: obesity, type 2 diabetes, cancer, endometriosis, polycystic ovary syndrome (PCOS), infertility, cardiovascular disease (CVD) and impact cognitive function. So, what could a healthy microbiome and active estrobolome do for us? With a healthy, diverse gut microbiome, the estrobolome can continue to make oestrogens available again and contribute to alleviating menopausal symptoms. In the long term, a healthy and diverse gut microbiome can help to reduce the risk of heart disease and other metabolic disease risk. Many women turn to eating phytoestrogen-rich foods such as tofu, soy and edamame beans.

Eating foods that contain isoflavones has been associated with reducing hot flushes and other symptoms experienced during menopause, as well as potentially reducing bone loss in the spine and lowering blood pressure[48]. While these foods are a helpful addition to our diets during perimenopause and menopause, the benefits of a diverse microbiome can only be reaped with a diet rich in a variety of plants. It's key to include plenty of diverse plant fibres and enjoy probiotic (fermented) foods before focusing too much on phytoestrogen-rich food consumption alone.

The best foods to accompany the menopausal transition are those rich in diversity of fibre and polyphenols, the colourful chemicals found in foods, which basically means lots of colourful plants. Throughout perimenopause and menopause, increasing the amount of

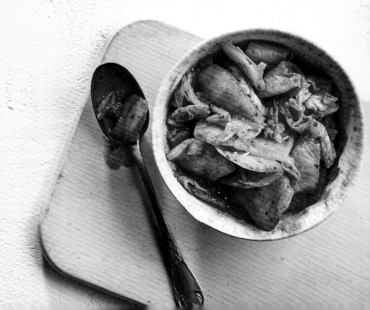

polyphenol-rich berries and dark green vegetables, as well as fibre-rich nuts, pulses and seeds, you eat can significantly improve all of the symptoms of menopause and decrease the risk of associated post-menopausal disease. Studies looking at simple interventions such as adding the equivalent of one cup of blueberries to your daily diet have shown significant improvements for markers of heart health and blood pressure[49], making adding these foods to your weekly shop an easy win for current and for future health.

When compared to diets rich in sweets, solid fats and snacks, having a diet rich in fruits and vegetables is clearly associated with better outcomes for our brains and bodies. Another element to focus on is the introduction of probiotic foods to our everyday diets. These foods aren't expensive supplements, they are traditional fermented foods and include plain natural yogurt, some cheeses and foods such as sauerkraut, kefir, miso and unsweetened kombucha. There are plenty of foods that can introduce new microbes every day, and hence increase microbial diversity to ensure our microbiome remains dynamic and rich in helpful strains.

PRE- PRO- POST- PARA- AND SYNBIOTIC: WHAT'S THE DEAL?

I've mentioned that the gut microbiome produces helpful chemicals, including the enzymes that free oestrogen back into the circulation. These helpful chemicals that are like a private pharmacy for our bodies are called metabolites or 'postbiotics'. If we look at the chain production of postbiotics step by step, it looks a little bit like this:

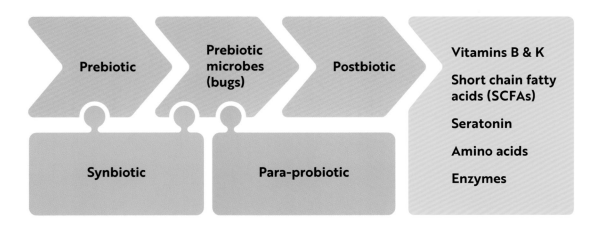

So prebiotic fibres are found in pretty much every single plant we eat, and increasing the variety of these prebiotic fibres leads to a more diverse microbe population. This is because each gut microbe prefers to use a specific type of fibre – the microbes that love apple don't necessarily love cucumber, and those that love artichokes can't do much good with spinach. Scientists are still working to understand exactly how individual foods impact gut microbiome composition in the long term.

When compared to diets rich in sweets, solid fats and snacks, having a diet rich in fruits and vegetables is clearly associated with better outcomes for our brains and bodies.

We know from some exciting studies that the gut microbiome can be changed quite significantly with the introduction of specific foods. One such study showed that a single dose of mixed curry spices can significantly impact gut microbiome composition[50], kimchi can help reduce obesity and drinking coffee (which is fermented coffee beans) is associated with lower risk of depression[51] all by modulating the gut microbiome. Synbiotic foods are foods like sauerkraut and kimchi[52], which contain both the prebiotic fibres and the live probiotic microbes. Some supplements call themselves synbiotic but really fermented foods are nature's synbiotics. Para-probiotics is a fairly new category which refers to the potential impact that even dead microbes can have on health. These might be microbes that have been killed due to heating and cooking, for example if we cook miso. It's still too early to know how much of an impact these might have but they are quite exciting for people who have a more compromised immune system and might be wary of consuming fermented food.

Every time a gut bug breaks down a prebiotic fibre, they make something for our bodies to use. These are called postbiotics and they are absolutely crucial for good health. Vitamins, neurotransmitters and even antimicrobial peptides that help kill bad bacteria are all produced by our gut microbes, and short chain fatty acids (SCFAs) such as butyrate help to keep our gut wall lining intact, stopping any unwanted pathogens and waste products from crossing the gut wall lining into the lymph system around our gut. Our gut wall is a single cell thick and held together by 'tight junctions' which don't allow unwanted cells to pass. These tight junctions need SCFAs to stay strong and if our gut health is disrupted, they can loosen and become less effective at keeping what's inside the gut from leaking out through the lining. When our gut microbes can't make enough SCFAs, our gut can become more permeable, sometimes referred to as 'leaky gut'. Severe malnutrition and recurring infection in malnourished children is where we see the most extreme examples of a compromised wall lining and leaky gut, leaving them vulnerable to infection and further malnutrition. In adults in countries like the UK and the US, the much less severe forms of leaky gut are associated with increased likelihood of allergies and intolerances, a weakened immune system and irritable bowel symptoms. All this shows just how important it is that we maintain a diverse and healthy microbiome. Eating lots of plants, keeping active throughout the day and giving our gut microbes a rest overnight are three simple steps to take to improve gut health.

It's worth noting here that unhelpful gut microbes travel through your body in the same way. For example, the production of TMAO (a metabolite produced by gut bacteria) is associated with a host of metabolic diseases including obesity, diabetes and high blood pressure. Eating too many animal foods such as beef, lamb, pork, veal and bacon results in higher levels of TMA reaching the gut and converted to TMAO by meat-loving gut bugs[53]. This is one of the reasons why we think that eating a lot of red meat over time can contribute to worse health outcomes in those people who have the meat-loving gut bugs. I want to be clear that this is different for everybody, and eating meat occasionally is unlikely to result in high levels of TMAO. I, and many women I work with, have removed red meat from our diets as we feel better without it. It's worth listening to your gut and removing foods that might cause the production of some of these unhelpful postbiotics.

THE GUT–BRAIN AXIS – FOOD FOR THOUGHT

Another important and now well-established role of the gut microbiome is its role in the gut–brain axis, a topic which deserves a book all of its own! The gut–brain axis is the most powerful connection that we know of, thanks to the direct link from gut to brain through the vagus nerve. The vagus nerve is the longest cranial (head) nerve and also connects the brain with the heart, liver and lungs. Anxiety is a mental health condition which is greatly influenced by our gut health, with research showing that certain dietary patterns increase the risk of developing anxiety and also make managing anxiety more difficult. On the flipside, we can use this knowledge to prevent and help treat anxiety through the food choices we make.

• The mighty microbiome •

Some people may suffer anxiety symptoms first, which then impact their food choices, others may find that when their diet changes, they suffer with anxiety. Gastrointestinal symptoms associated with anxiety vary widely and include bloating, flatulence, loose stools and constipation. Irritable Bowel Syndrome (IBS) is associated with anxiety, and they are typically closely linked.

We have enough evidence now to say that increasing whole plant foods such as vegetables, beans and pulses, nuts and whole fruits has a significant impact on symptoms of anxiety. Reviews have shown the beneficial impact of Mediterranean Diet patterns on our brains, and this fits in with our knowledge of the microbiome and gut–brain axis.

To get as much plant variety as possible, try eating seasonally to taste new vegetables and fruits, as well as adding nuts and seeds to your salads or yogurt and using herbs and spices in cooking. Polyphenol-rich foods like berries and extra virgin olive oil should be part of our everyday diet, and we should aim to consume probiotic foods like kefir, kombucha or sauerkraut every day too. Deep breathing exercises are also really helpful in stimulating the vagus nerve to reduce anxiety and stress, so there is a lot of evidence to support mindfulness and breathwork in easing anxiety symptoms.

When anxiety is severe and impeding social function, it's advisable to ask for psychotherapeutic support, which is proven to work better than medication in the long term, so alongside changes in nutrition and lifestyle – breathwork and exercise, for example – it is sometimes necessary to ask for help which is effective and can make a huge difference.

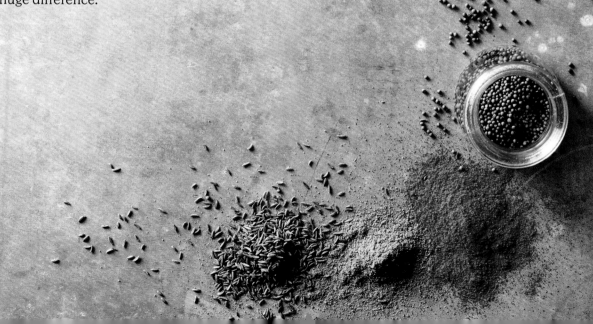

Foods for the menopause transition: from first symptoms to post-menopause

Understanding how and why our changing bodies react to food differently as we go through menopause is the first step in being able to improve the journey. Now we've seen how our microbiome changes, how oestrogen levels can impact our food choices, how our bodies change the way they store fat and how our mental health changes during menopause. We also know that after menopause we are at a higher risk of certain diseases, but that these risks can be mitigated by diet and we can use this pivotal point in our lives to focus on ourselves, our health and our longevity.

A recent review concluded that over 50% of women seek complementary solutions to managing menopausal symptoms. HRT is not for everyone and it's not a magic bullet, so thinking holistically is really important. With one out of three women currently estimated to be perimenopausal or post-menopausal right now, it makes sense to highlight the practical, effective solutions and changes we can make.

From night sweats to changes in skin texture, the table opposite recaps the evidence of what we can do to support our bodies and our minds. Vasomotor symptoms such as hot flushes are experienced by up to 90% of perimenopausal women over 4–10 years before menopause. Vasomotor symptoms are closely linked with smoking, excess body fat and alcohol, for example. A Mediterranean Diet is associated with a reduction in vasomotor symptoms and improved mental health outcomes, as well as better chances of healthy weight management.

Diet and joint pain are more manageable with a healthier weight, and we can also be quite sure that supplements such as red clover and black cohosh do not have a significant impact on symptoms. Isoflavones from soy foods don't have a huge impact but they are healthy foods to enjoy, and there is some evidence that collagen supplementing could improve skin texture. Finally, multivitamin supplements, vitamin D and fish oils don't have an impact whereas a diet rich in lots of vitamins from plants and whole oily fish does.

Early Perimenopause

Later Perimenopause

Fatigue

Shortened menstrual cycle

Anxiety

Vaginal dryness

Overwhelm

Difficulty coping

Pelvic floor issues

Nocturia
(waking in the night because you need to urinate)

Weight gain

Loss of libido

Night sweats

Hot flushes

Erratic periods

Vaginal atrophy

Menopause-Friendly Foods: Eat and Avoid

Symptoms	System	Try this	Avoid this
Hot flushes	Vasomotor	Blueberries, beetroot, cavolo nero, cauliflower	Alcohol, spicy food
Night sweats	Vasomotor	Dark fruits like plums, blackberries and blueberries	Alcohol, late meals
Heart palpitations	Hormonal	Tofu, edamame, breathing exercises	Coffee, added sugars, biscuits and packaged snacks
Anxiety	Mental health	Salmon, mackerel, whole grains, seasonal vegetables, mushrooms	Ultra-processed foods, sugar-free and low-fat desserts
Vaginal dryness	Hormonal	Extra virgin olive oil, topical oestrogen, lubricant	Refined carbohydrates, fizzy drinks, intimate soaps
Fat weight gain	Hormonal	Dark leafy greens, beans and legumes, chicken, tofu and mushrooms	Ultra-processed foods, refined carbohydrates
Poor sleep	Hormonal	Natural yogurt, kiwi fruit, maintain a consistent sleep window	Alcohol, spicy foods

Symptoms	System	Try this	Avoid this
Stiff joints	Inflammation	Fresh spices, oily fish, extra virgin olive oil	Refined carbohydrates, alcohol
Loss of sense of self	Mental health	Mushrooms, nuts, chickpeas, barley	Ultra-processed foods, alcohol
Mood changes	Mental health	Dark fruits like plums, dark leafy vegetables	Ultra-processed foods, alcohol
Brain fog	Cognitive	Beetroot, dark chocolate, mushrooms, cherries and raspberries	Refined carbohydrates (e.g. white bread and pastries)
Skin changes	Inflammation	Berries, dark leafy greens, chickpeas, collagen supplementation	Alcohol, ultra-processed foods
Overwhelm	Mental health	Lentils, beans, tofu, chicken, nuts	Caffeine, alcohol, refined carbohydrates
Weight gain	Hormonal and metabolic	Eggs, beans, broccoli, mushrooms, green leafy veg, natural yogurt, barley	Ultra-processed foods, refined carbohydrates, alcohol, late-night snacks
Changes in frequency and urgency of urination	Hormonal	Dark leafy greens, dark berries, red cabbage	Alcohol, not drinking enough water

List of Foods

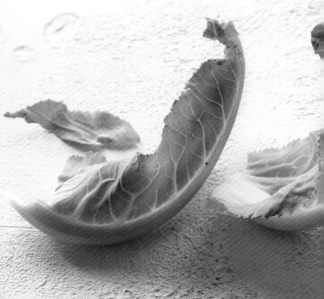

Always	Regularly
Extra virgin olive oil	Tofu
Kale	Edamame
Cavolo nero	Salmon/trout/mackerel
Barley	A glass of red wine
Buckwheat	Apples
Spelt	Pears
Berries	Eggs
Fermented foods	Natural yogurt
(kraut, kimchi, kefir)	Dark chocolate (70%+)
Spices	Kombucha
Herbs	Sweet potato/white potato
Avocado	Nut butters
Rocket	Banana 'nice' cream
Peppers	Chicken
Spinach	Spelt pasta
Mushrooms	Seeded dark rye sourdough
Nuts	All whole fruits
Seeds	
Chickpeas	
Lentils	
Beans	
Dark fruits like plums	
Dr Fede's spice mix (page 180)	
Broccoli/cauliflower	
Cabbages	
Peas and other frozen veg	
Coffee or green tea	
Gram flour wraps	
All whole vegetables	

Occasionally

Red meat
Potato crisps
Home-baked cakes and pastries
Other wine/beer
White rice
White pasta

Rarely

Cakes
Pastries
Doughnuts
Sugary drinks
Ice cream
Biscuits
Processed meats
Ultra-processed foods
Sweets

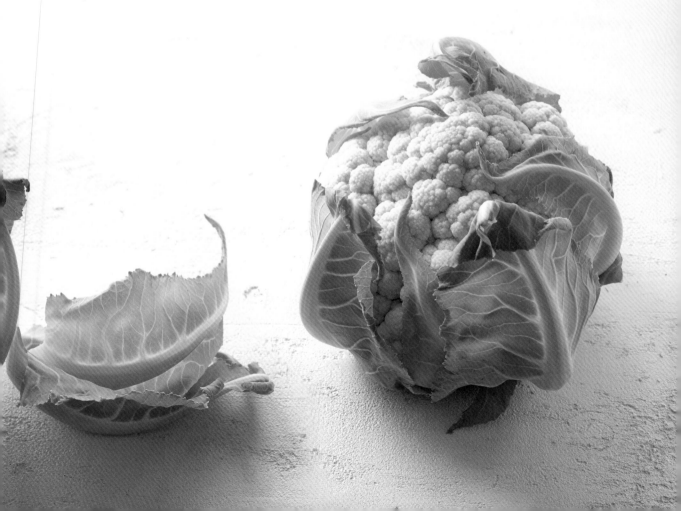

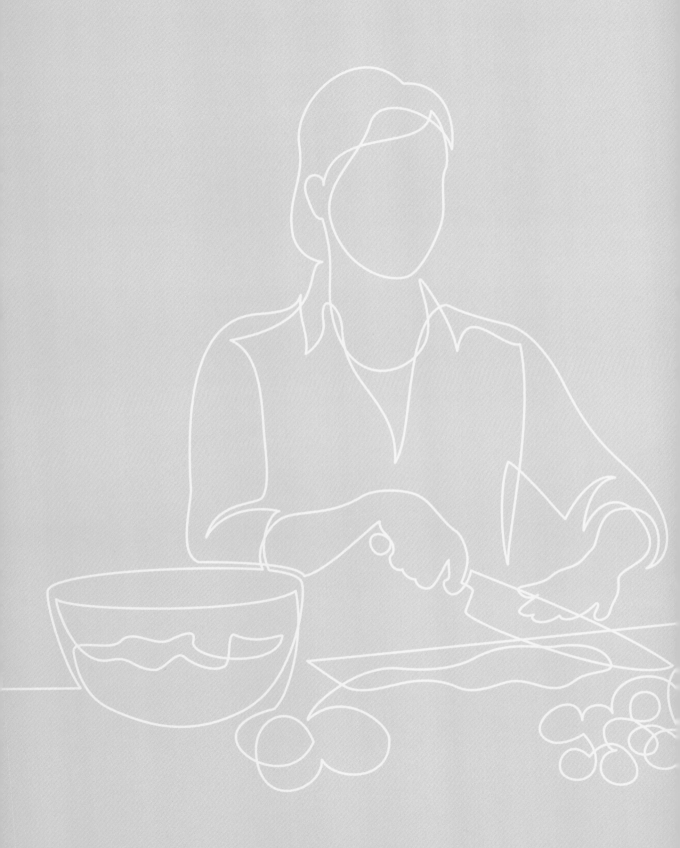

Recipes

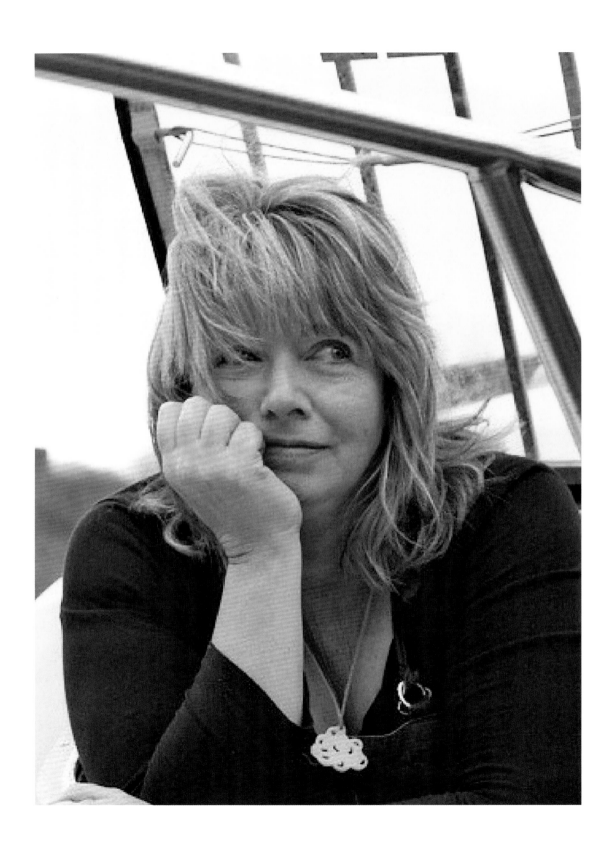

Introduction by Jane Baxter

As you embark on your menopause journey, the Mediterranean Diet can be a valuable ally. Drawing on my experience of cooking plant-based meals with a southern Italian influence for many years, it provided an excellent starting point when it came to catering for the changes in my own body.

As a new mother in my forties, I never imagined that my child's teenage years would coincide with my transition through menopause, which was compounded by the stresses of launching a new business. These life changes prompted me to take a closer look at my diet and physical wellbeing. In this recipe book, I've gathered a collection of tried-and-tested recipes, incorporating Dr Federica's research and ingredients known to ease menopausal symptoms.

My goal is to offer dishes that are both delicious and achievable. This isn't a book about maintaining a certain appearance or losing weight, although it may have those benefits. Rather, I hope it will help you rediscover the pleasure of eating during menopause and beyond, making it a joy rather than a chore.

Breakfast

1

Mexican eggs

The green sauce in the mushroom recipe (page 96) can also be drizzled over this dish. The peperonata base is a good side to serve with grilled fish or meat as well as with the eggs, and can also be made in advance and reheated when you are ready to cook with eggs.

Serves 4

400g (14oz) can black beans, drained

4 eggs

1 avocado

juice of 1 lime

2 tablespoons chopped coriander

70g (2½oz) feta

Peperonata base

3 tablespoons olive oil

1 large onion, finely sliced

3 peppers (a mix of red, orange and yellow if possible), deseeded and finely sliced

3 garlic cloves, crushed

400g (14oz) can chopped tomatoes or passata

pinch of cayenne pepper, ground cumin and dried oregano

1 tablespoon balsamic vinegar

salt and pepper

1 To make the peperonata base, heat the olive oil in a large frying pan and tip in the sliced onion. Season with salt and cook gently for 20 minutes without browning. Add the peppers and stir well. Cook for a further 20 minutes until the peppers have softened.

2 Add the garlic and cook for 2 minutes, then tip in the chopped tomatoes along with the spices and oregano. Stir well and simmer gently for another 20 minutes until the tomatoes have reduced and are coating the peppers. Season well and add the balsamic vinegar.

3 Add the black beans to the peperonata. Cook for a few minutes to warm through.

4 Make 4 wells in the pan and crack an egg into each one. Cover the pan and cook gently for about 5 minutes or until the eggs are set to your liking.

5 Chop the avocado roughly and mix with the lime juice. Season well.

6 To serve, sprinkle the eggs with the avocado and coriander. Crumble the feta over the top to finish.

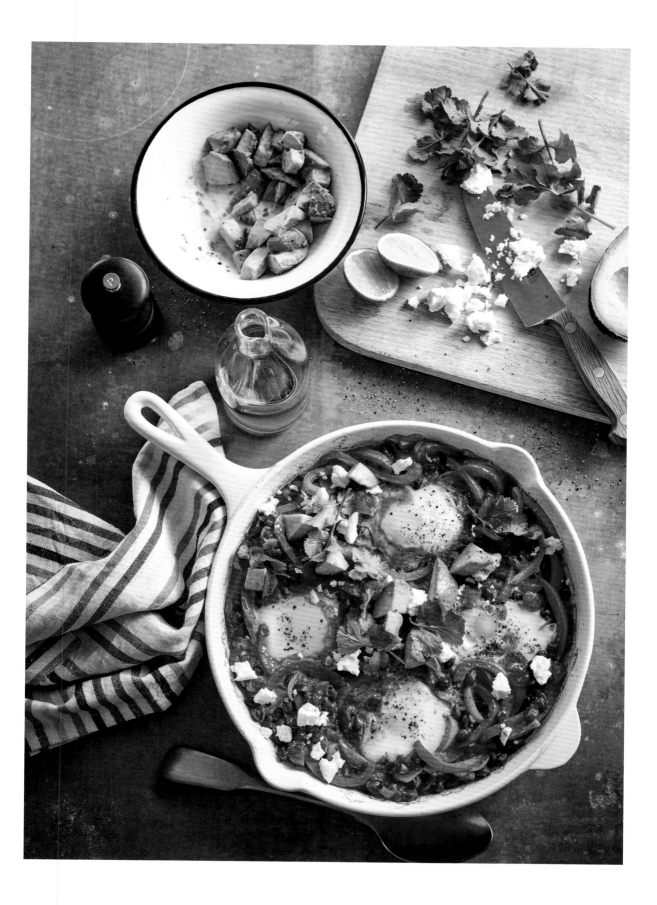

Overnight oats

A great option for breakfast. The oats will keep in the fridge for 4 days after soaking. Serve as they are or with any of the suggested toppings.

Serves 2

Base

50g (1¾oz) steel-cut whole oats (organic where possible)

125ml (4fl oz) kefir

125ml (4fl oz) oat milk (or milk of choice) or water

1 tablespoon chia seeds

1 apple or pear, peeled and grated

handful of almonds or macadamia nuts

Toppings (optional)

peanut butter or toasted coconut

chopped dried apricots and walnuts

mixed berries (frozen or fresh) and pumpkin seeds

grated carrot, toasted coconut, toasted walnuts, cinnamon and sultanas

1 Mix the oats with the rest of the base ingredients. Mix well and place in a glass bowl or Kilner jar, cover and leave in the fridge for at least 6 hours or overnight.

2 Top with the topping of your choice, if you like.

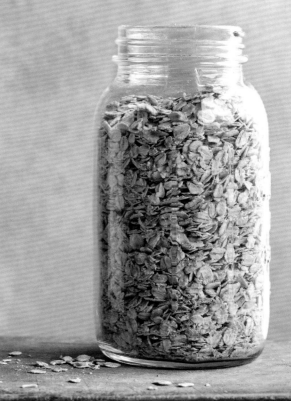

Methi dhal with fried eggs

Moong dhal is traditionally used in this recipe but if it is hard to come by it's fine to substitute split yellow peas or red lentils. Methi leaves can be bought online or in Indian supermarkets, though spinach, kale or chard can be used instead, along with celery leaves or watercress leaves. Raita (page 176) and Kachumber (page 118) are perfect accompaniments. Ikan bilis (dried anchovies) and peanuts fried together add texture and amazing flavour, plus extra protein.

Serves 4

200g (7oz) moong dhal

2 teaspoons grated fresh ginger

½ teaspoon ground turmeric

1 tablespoon coconut oil

1 teaspoon black mustard seeds

1 teaspoon cumin seeds

1 sprig of fresh curry leaves, leaves picked

pinch of chilli flakes

1 green chilli, deseeded and chopped (optional)

1 teaspoon dried fenugreek leaves

pinch of asafoetida

1 onion, chopped

4 tomatoes, chopped

3 garlic cloves, crushed

1 teaspoon salt

2 bunches of fresh fenugreek (methi) leaves

1 teaspoon garam masala

4 fried eggs, to serve

1 Rinse the lentils in lots of cold running water. Place in a pan with about 750ml (1⅓ pints) water, the grated ginger and turmeric. Bring to the boil and simmer for about 30 minutes or until the lentils are very soft. Season with salt and pepper. Set aside.

2 In a large, shallow pan, heat the coconut oil and add the mustard and cumin seeds, curry leaves, chilli flakes, fresh chilli (if using) and dried fenugreek. Cook for a few minutes over a high heat, stirring well, until the mustard seeds start to pop.

3 Add the asafoetida and chopped onion and cook over a low heat for about 5 minutes, then add the tomatoes, 1 teaspoon of salt and the garlic. Simmer for 10 minutes.

4 Wash and roughly chop the methi leaves and add them to the tomato base. Cook until wilted, then tip into the dhal. At this point, add extra water to the dhal if you prefer it to be not too thick. Simmer for 5 minutes, check the seasoning and stir through the garam masala.

5 Serve each portion topped with a fried egg.

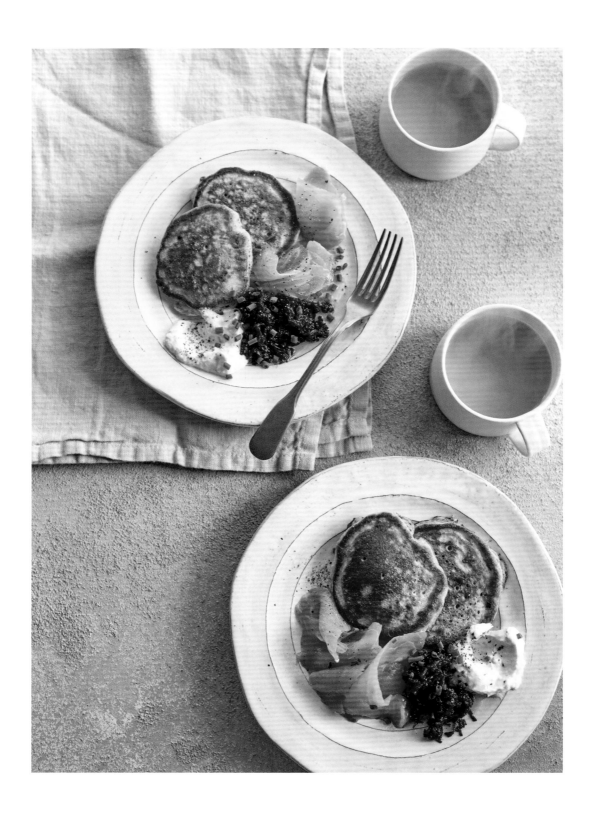

Buckwheat & sauerkraut pancakes with salmon

A versatile pancake batter. The sauerkraut can be swapped for kimchi, with coriander and spring onions added instead of the herbs.

Serves 4

4 eggs, separated

250ml (9fl oz) kefir

100g (3½oz) buckwheat flour

100g (3½oz) spelt flour

1 tablespoon honey

½ teaspoon baking powder

½ teaspoon bicarbonate of soda

2 teaspoons caraway seeds

3 tablespoons chopped sauerkraut

1 tablespoon chopped chives

1 tablespoon chopped dill

50ml (2fl oz) olive oil, for frying

salt and pepper

Toppings (optional)

Raita or beetroot raita (page 176)

smoked salmon and poached eggs

salmon with grated beetroot and horseradish

1 Whisk the egg yolks with the kefir, flours and honey until you have a smooth batter.

2 Whisk the egg whites to soft peaks and fold into the batter. Gently fold in the remaining ingredients, except the oil, with salt and pepper to taste.

3 Make the pancakes in batches. Start by heating half the oil in a non-stick frying pan and add a tablespoon of the batter for each pancake. Cook over a medium heat for 2 minutes, then flip the pancakes over and cook for another 2 minutes. Transfer the pancakes to a very low oven to keep warm and repeat with the rest of the oil until all the batter is used up.

4 Serve with the toppings of your choice, if you like.

Fermented foods like sauerkraut are full of probiotic live bacteria, excellent for gut health.

Quinoa pancakes with green sauce & mushrooms

These crisp quinoa pancakes can also be used alongside many other dishes or dips.

Serves 4

Quinoa pancakes

250g (9oz) cooked quinoa

1 carrot, peeled and grated

1 red onion, grated

2 eggs

2 tablespoons sesame seeds

1 tablespoon chopped chives

1 tablespoon chickpea flour

olive oil, for frying and drizzling

salt and pepper to serve

Green sauce

1 green chilli

1 tablespoon chopped flat leaf parsley

1 tablespoon chopped coriander

1 tablespoon chopped mint

2 garlic cloves, crushed

juice of ½ lemon

50ml (2fl oz) olive oil

120g (4¼oz) tahini

2 tablespoons Greek yogurt

Mushrooms

2 tablespoons olive oil

400g (14oz) mixed mushrooms, sliced

2 garlic cloves, crushed

1 In a small bowl, mix all the quinoa pancake ingredients, except the oil, together until well combined and season well.

2 Place all the green sauce ingredients in a blender and mix until smooth, adding a little water to the sauce until it's the consistency of lightly whipped cream.

3 Heat the oil for the mushrooms in a large frying pan, tip in the mushrooms and garlic, and cook until the mushrooms have wilted, seasoning only when they are tender.

4 Make the pancakes in batches. In a small non-stick frying pan, heat 2 tablespoons of olive oil and spoon in a heaped tablespoon of the batter per pancake, frying for a few minutes on each side until crisp. Repeat for the next batch until all the batter is used up.

5 Serve the green sauce topped with the mushrooms, with the pancakes on the side.

Quinoa is one of the most nutrient-rich grains and a great source of protein, containing all nine essential amino acids.

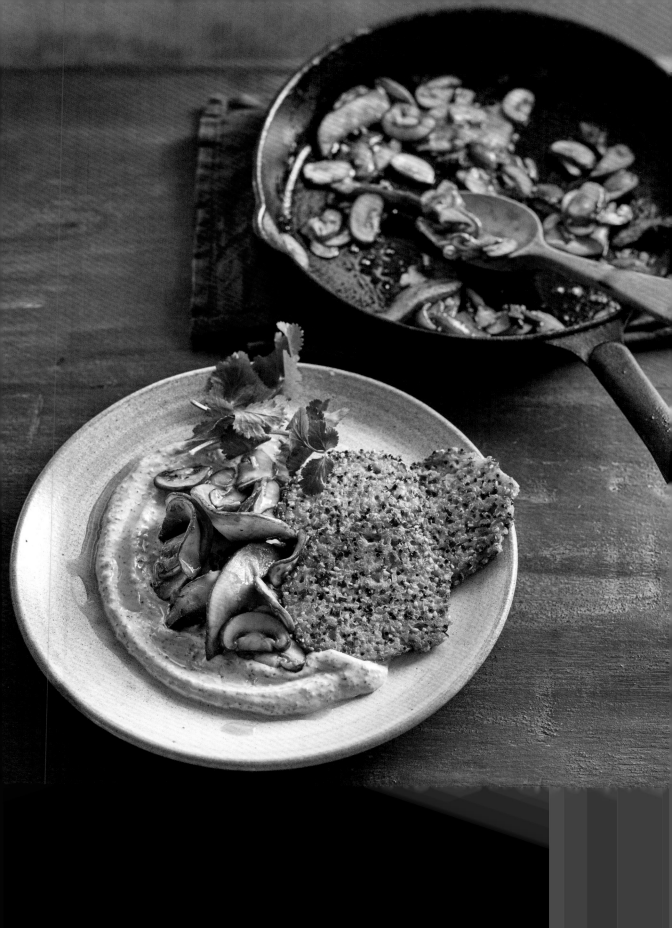

Scrambled tofu

Any green vegetables can be used in this recipe such as cooked spinach, French beans or sugar snap peas.

Serves 4

2 tablespoons olive oil

1 red onion, finely chopped

1 red pepper, deseeded and finely chopped

1 chilli, deseeded and chopped

1 garlic clove, crushed

½ teaspoon ground turmeric

pinch of ground cumin and coriander

200g (7oz) small broccoli and cauliflower florets

100g (3½oz) frozen peas

6 cherry tomatoes, halved

300g (10½oz) medium or firm tofu

2 tablespoons soy sauce

1 bunch of spring onions, chopped

1 tablespoon chopped coriander

salt and pepper

1 Heat the oil in a shallow frying pan and add the chopped onion and red pepper. Cook over a medium heat for about 10 minutes until softened. Add the chilli, garlic and spices. Cook for a further few minutes and stir well.

2 Add the vegetables, cover the pan and allow to steam over a gentle heat for about 5 minutes or until just cooked.

3 Stir through the tomatoes and crumble the tofu into the pan. Fold through the vegetables and sprinkle with the soy sauce. Cook for a few minutes longer before sprinkling with the spring onions and coriander. Season well.

Miso eggs & tomatoes

A classic Chinese dish with added miso, which can also be served as a side. Protein-rich foods are great for our metabolism, and adding miso is brilliant for gut health.

Serves 4

25g (1oz) salted butter, softened

50ml (2fl oz) olive oil

2 tablespoons white miso paste

6 eggs

1 teaspoon sesame oil

2 teaspoons Shaoxing wine

6 spring onions, chopped

4 tomatoes, each cut into 6 wedges

pinch of brown sugar

1 tablespoon light soy sauce

1 tablespoon toasted sesame seeds (or seed mix, page 181)

black pepper

1 Beat together the butter, olive oil and miso until well combined.

2 Beat the eggs with the sesame oil, wine and 1 tablespoon of water and season with pepper.

3 In a large, shallow non-stick pan, warm the miso mixture over a low heat. Turn up the heat and tip in the eggs, folding carefully for a few minutes until they are just cooked and coated with the miso. Scoop out of the pan into a bowl.

4 Add the spring onions to the pan and fry for a few minutes. Tip in the tomatoes with the sugar and cook over a medium heat for about 10 minutes or until they have softened. Return the eggs to the pan, stir in the soy sauce and fold into the tomatoes. Cook for another 2 minutes and serve with a sprinkling of seeds.

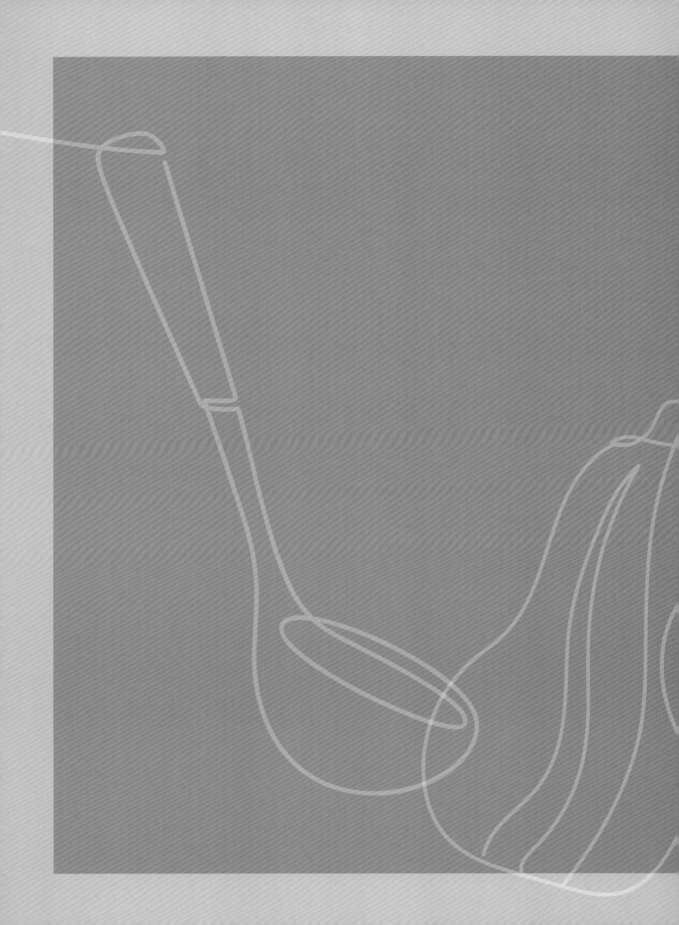

Spring minestrone

Frozen peas and broad beans are more than acceptable to use in this soup.

Serves 6

3 tablespoons olive oil

1 onion, finely chopped

1 leek, finely chopped

2 celery sticks, finely chopped

3 garlic cloves, crushed

1 Parmesan rind, plus 2 tablespoons grated Parmesan

300g (10½oz) courgettes, diced

150g (5½oz) broad beans (fresh or frozen)

200g (7oz) asparagus, chopped into 1–2cm (½–¾in) pieces

100g (3½oz) sugar snap peas, sliced

100g (3½oz) peas (fresh or frozen)

750ml (1⅓ pints) vegetable stock

2 tablespoons chopped basil

2 tablespoons chopped mint

6 spring onions, chopped

extra virgin olive oil, for drizzling

salt and pepper

1 Heat the oil in a large pan and gently cook the onion, leek and celery over a low heat for about 15 minutes without browning. Add the garlic and Parmesan rind and cook for another minute.

2 Stir in the courgettes and cook for about 10 minutes until almost tender. Add the broad beans and asparagus and cook for 5 minutes. Add the sugar snaps, peas and stock. Bring to a simmer and cook gently for 2 minutes.

3 Remove the cheese rind and season. Stir in the herbs and spring onions. Remove about a quarter of the soup and blitz in a food processor until smooth. Stir back into the soup. Season to taste. Serve drizzled with olive oil and sprinkled with grated Parmesan.

We often overlook onions, being so commonly used, but they contain inulin, a prebiotic that encourages healthy gut bacteria.

Squash, fennel & lentil soup

**The squash stock, using the seeds and trimmings,
can be used in other squash soups or stews.**

Serves 6

1 butternut squash

3 tablespoons olive oil

1 onion, finely chopped

2 heads of fennel, finely chopped

3 garlic cloves, crushed

pinch of chilli flakes

200g (7oz) Puy lentils (or green lentils)

salt and pepper

Squash stock

1 onion, halved

1 celery stick, halved

1 leek top

1 carrot

1 bay leaf

1 sprig of thyme

parsley stalks

1 Peel the squash, reserving the insides, seeds and trimmings but discarding the skin. Place all the trimmings and the seeds in a pan with the stock vegetables and any trimmings from the fennel. Cover with about 1 litre (1¾ pints) of water and simmer for 30 minutes. Drain and reserve the stock. Cut the squash into 1cm (½in) rough chunks and set aside.

2 In a large pan, cook the onion and fennel in the olive oil over a low heat for 10 minutes. Add the garlic and chilli flakes and cook for a minute. Stir in the lentils and squash pieces. Pour in the reserved stock and simmer for about 20 minutes or until the lentils and squash are cooked.

3 Blitz about a quarter of the soup in a food processor until smooth and return to the pan. Stir well to combine and season. Add water until you achieve your desired consistency.

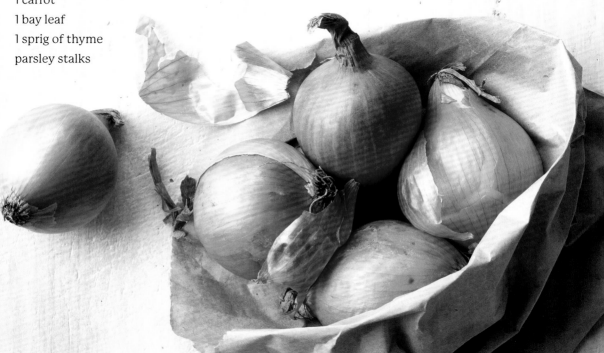

Seafood soup with kimchi & vegetables

This tasty and nutritious soup combines texture and flavour, making it a brilliant dish. It is high in protein, fibre, polyphenols, fermented foods, iron and omega-3s – a real all-rounder! It's worth searching for a good-quality kimchi for this dish. Other vegetables can be used in this soup – sugar snaps, French beans or pak choi could be substituted.

Serves 6

2 tablespoons olive oil

1 onion, chopped

2 garlic cloves, crushed

2cm (¾in) piece of fresh ginger, peeled and grated

2 tablespoons Korean gochujang paste

2 leeks, sliced

2 courgettes, diced

150g (5½oz) kimchi

500ml (18fl oz) fish sock

1 tablespoon light soy sauce

1 tablespoon fish sauce

1 tablespoon mirin

200g (7oz) raw prawns, shelled and deveined

500g (1lb 2oz) mussels, cleaned

100g (3½oz) squid, cleaned and sliced

300g (10½oz) silken tofu

100g (3½oz) beansprouts

Salt and pepper

1 In a large pan, heat the olive oil and cook the onion, garlic and ginger over a low heat for 5 minutes. Stir in the gochujang paste and cook for a minute before adding the vegetables and kimchi. Stir well and add the fish stock, soy and fish sauces, and mirin. Bring to a gentle boil and simmer for 5 minutes.

2 Add the prawns, mussels and squid to the seasoned stock. Cover and cook gently for 5 minutes or until the mussels have just opened. Cut the tofu into 1–2cm (½–¾in) squares and add to the soup along with the beansprouts.

3 Stir well and cook for another minute. Check the seasoning and serve.

Squid is a good source of vitamin B12 as well as potassium, iron, phosphorus and copper.

Salads

3

Myanmar fermented tea leaf salad

A good friend brought me some pickled tea leaves after a visit to Myanmar and mentioned their use in salads. There are lots of salad variations; some have dried prawns and other chopped vegetables. The leaves can be quite hard to find but equal amounts of chopped kimchi and sauerkraut can be used instead. I have increased the amounts of nuts and seeds in this recipe along with the fried split peas to give lots of texture to the salad.

Serves 6

75g (2½oz) dried split peas, soaked overnight in lots of cold water

50ml (2fl oz) olive oil

10 garlic cloves, finely sliced

50g (1¾oz) sunflower seeds, toasted

50g (1¾oz) pumpkin seeds, toasted

75g (2½oz) peanuts, toasted

2 tablespoons sesame seeds, toasted

200g (7oz) cabbage, finely sliced

2 heads of little gem, finely sliced

200g (7oz) cherry tomatoes, quartered

3–4 tablespoons fermented tea leaves (or a mixture of chopped sauerkraut and kimchi)

juice of ½ lime

1 tablespoon fish sauce

1 tablespoon light soy sauce

Salt and pepper

1 Drain the split peas and dry well. Heat the oil in a shallow frying pan and fry the split peas for 5 minutes until they are slightly brown and crisp. Remove with a slotted spoon onto kitchen paper. In the remaining oil, fry the garlic slices until they are just starting to brown.

2 Toss the browned split peas and garlic with the remaining ingredients. Taste and add more lime or seasoning if required.

Packed with powerful plant chemicals, cabbage is great for gut health and contributes to a healthy heart.

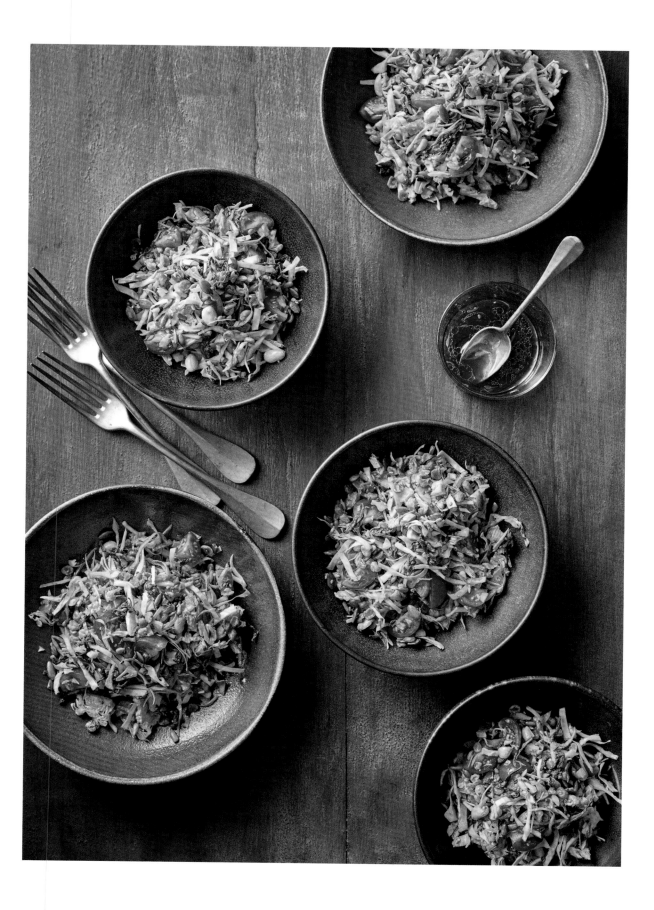

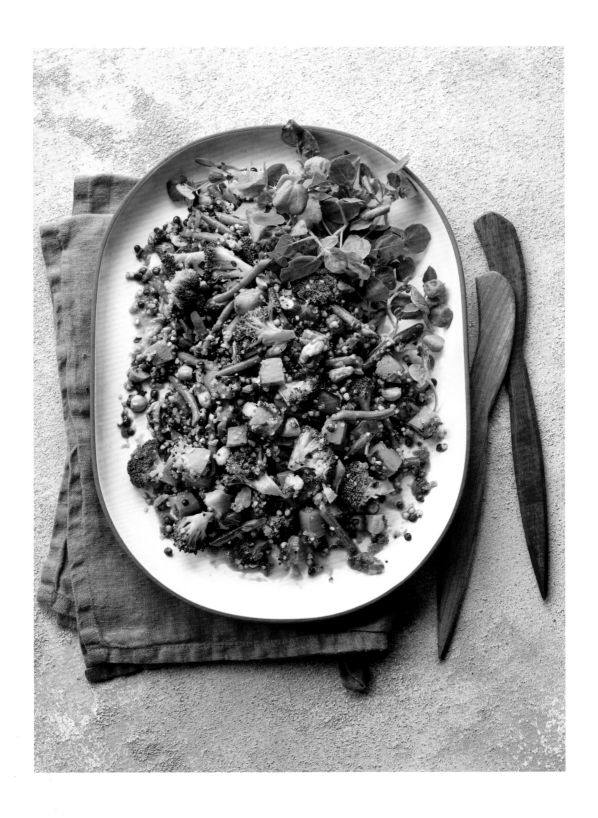

Squash, greens & nut salad with a ginger dressing

This salad is a good way to use up cooked grains. Any other green vegetables can be used – whatever you have to hand or is in season. Top with some mixed seeds (page 181) for added protein.

Serves 6

200g (7oz) butternut squash, peeled and cut into 1–2cm (½–¾in) dice

3 tablespoons olive oil

100g (3½oz) broccoli florets

100g (3½oz) French beans, trimmed

150g (5½oz) mixed nuts (cashews, almonds and pecans), toasted

100g (3½oz) cooked Puy lentils

100g (3½oz) cooked quinoa

100g (3½oz) cooked buckwheat

2 tablespoons chopped chives

1 bunch of watercress

salt and pepper

Dressing

75ml (2½fl oz) honey

50ml (2fl oz) rice vinegar

1 tablespoon mirin

50ml (2fl oz) light soy sauce

2cm (¾in) piece of fresh ginger, peeled and grated

1 garlic clove, crushed

1 tablespoon pickled ginger, chopped

1 Preheat the oven to 160°C (325°F/gas mark 3).

2 Toss the squash pieces in 1 tablespoon of olive oil and season. Tip on a baking tray and roast for about 20 minutes or until just tender.

3 Blanch the broccoli and beans seperately until just cooked. Refresh under cold running water and drain. Roughly chop the nuts and place in a large bowl with the squash, broccoli, beans and cooked lentils and grains. Season well and fold together with the remaining olive oil.

4 Whisk all the dressing ingredients together and drizzle over the salad. Arrange the salad on a serving dish. Sprinkle with the chives and place the watercress around the dish.

Ginger is rich in plant chemicals and helps with symptoms of heartburn and nausea as well as reducing inflammation.

Kachumber

A fabulous side with an Indian curry or as a salad on its own. Adding a little balsamic vinegar is not traditional but it really works. Toasting the cumin seeds before grinding is worth the effort for the best flavour.

Serves 4

300g (10½oz) cherry tomatoes, quartered

½ cucumber peeled, deseeded and cut into 1cm (½in) chunks

2 small red onions, finely chopped

2 tablespoons balsamic vinegar

2 teaspoons light soft brown sugar

1 garlic clove, crushed

2 teaspoons cumin seeds, toasted and ground

2 tablespoons shredded mint

1 tablespoon chopped coriander

salt and pepper

1 Place the tomatoes in a bowl with the cucumber pieces. Mix the onions with the vinegar, sugar and garlic. Mix well and allow to sit for at least 10 minutes.

2 Add the onion to the tomatoes and cucumber along with the remaining ingredients, stir and season. Best served immediately but will keep for a day in the fridge.

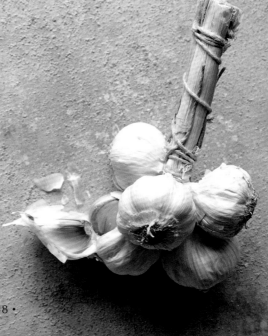

Tuna, white beans & celery

A classic Italian salad that's very quick to make.

Serves 4

3 celery sticks with leaves, cut into 1cm (½in) rough dice

1 red onion, finely chopped

250g (9oz) cannellini beans (canned or cooked from dried beans)

120g (4¼oz) canned tuna, drained

2 garlic cloves, crushed

1 tablespoon red wine vinegar

3 tablespoons olive oil

3 tablespoons chopped flat leaf parsley

1 tablespoon chopped chives

2 tablespoons capers (salted or in vinegar), rinsed

4 radishes, thinly sliced

extra virgin olive oil, for drizzling

salt and pepper

1 Fold all the ingredients together in a large bowl.

2 Season and serve drizzled with a little oil.

Cannellini beans are high in fibre, protein and flavour as well as being packed full of B vitamins essential for healthy brain function and metabolism.

Iceberg cups with spicy coleslaw & peanut sauce

Omit the chicken and shrimp paste for a vegetarian version, swapping the fish sauce for tamarind.

Serves 4

½ hispi cabbage

½ red pepper

1 shallot

2 carrots, peeled

1 apple

50g (1¾oz) French beans

1 red chilli

200g (7oz) cooked chicken, shredded

2 tablespoons chopped coriander

juice of 1 lime

1 tablespoon light soft brown sugar

1 tablespoon fish sauce

1 iceberg lettuce

Peanut sauce

1 shallot, chopped

1 tablespoon chopped lemongrass

½ teaspoon shrimp paste

large pinch of cayenne pepper, ground cumin
   and coriander

2 garlic cloves, crushed

250ml (9fl oz) coconut milk

1 tablespoon coconut oil

150g (5½oz) roasted peanuts, ground
   (or crunchy peanut butter)

2 tablespoons light soft brown sugar

1 tablespoon fish sauce

salt

1 Using a blender, make a paste with the shallot, lemongrass, shrimp paste, spices and garlic. Add a little of the coconut milk if necessary. Heat the coconut oil in a pan and gently cook the paste for 5 minutes until fragrant. Add the remaining coconut milk and simmer for a few minutes, mixing well.

2 Add the peanuts, sugar and fish sauce and simmer gently for another few minutes. Season with salt. If the sauce is too thick, let it down with a little water.

3 Finely shred the cabbage, red pepper and shallot. Grate the carrots and apple. Finely slice the French beans and chilli. Mix in a large bowl with the chicken and coriander.

4 Mix together the lime juice, sugar and fish sauce. Toss with the salad.

5 Cut the lettuce in half and gently separate the leaves to make the iceberg cups. Fill each cup with a little slaw and drizzle with a little peanut sauce. Any leftover sauce is lovely with grilled chicken or vegetables.

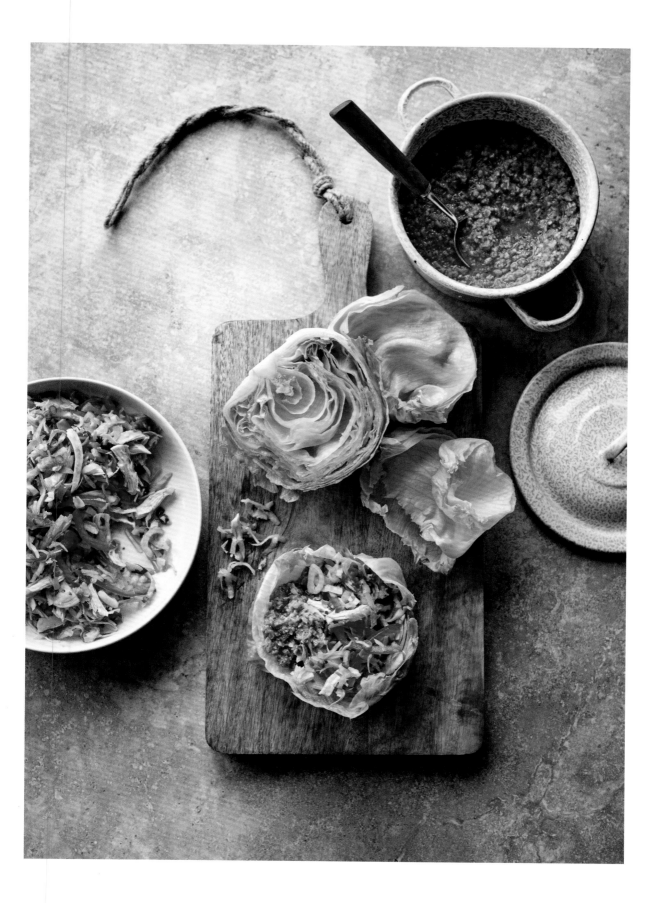

Truffled farro, turkey, mushrooms & peas

Farro is used quite a lot in Italy for salads and this is a version of an Umbrian dish. Cooked farro can also be combined with a classic basil pesto and grilled Mediterranean vegetables.

Serves 6

200g (7oz) farro
750ml (1⅓ pints) chicken stock
truffle oil
75ml (2½fl oz) olive oil
300g (10½oz) minced turkey
250g (9oz) mushrooms, sliced
2 garlic cloves, crushed
200g (7oz) frozen peas
1 tablespoon chopped tarragon
1 tablespoon chopped chives
2 tablespoons kefir yogurt
salt and pepper

1 Rinse the farro in cold running water. Place in a pan with the chicken stock and a pinch of salt. Bring to the boil and simmer over a low heat for about 25 minutes until the farro is tender but still has a little bite. Drain and season with a little truffle oil. Place in a large bowl.

2 In a large non-stick frying pan, heat half the olive oil and stir-fry the turkey for about 10 minutes until cooked through. Season and tip into the bowl with the farro.

3 Heat the remaining oil in the same pan, then add the sliced mushrooms and the garlic. Cook over a medium heat for 10 minutes until the mushrooms are tender. Season and add to bowl.

4 Cook the peas in boiling salted water for a minute. Drain and add to the farro. Allow to cool a little and fold together. Add the herbs and kefir yoghurt. Stir and drizzle with truffle oil.

Mixed bean, feta, herb & quinoa salad

Frozen peas, broad beans and edamame are perfect for this dish.

Serves 6

75g (2½oz) edamame

75g (2½oz) peas

75g (2½oz) broad beans

75g (2½oz) runner beans, thinly sliced

75g (2½oz) French beans, sliced into 1cm (½in) pieces

75g (2½oz) sugar snap peas, sliced

150g (5½oz) cooked quinoa

100g (3½oz) feta, crumbled

Dressing

1 garlic clove, crushed

2 tablespoons moscatel vinegar

4 tablespoons olive oil

2 teaspoons maple syrup

1 tablespoon chopped dill

1 tablespoon chopped mint

1 tablespoon chopped flat leaf parsley

1 tablespoon chopped tarragon

salt and pepper

1 Whisk all the dressing ingredients together in a large bowl and season.

2 In a large pot of boiling salted water, cook the beans and peas in separate batches until just cooked. After each batch, scoop out the beans or peas with a slotted spoon, drain and tip straight into the dressing. When all the beans and peas are cooked, stir through the quinoa and season.

3 Serve the salad with the feta crumbled on top.

Edamame contain isoflavones, which could help some women with their menopausal symptoms. Their high-fibre content is great for our gut microbiome.

Rocket salad with Parmesan & walnuts

A great salad to start any meal. The walnuts add protein and fibre. The rocket and lollo rosso are rich in polyphenols and the dressing is delicious.

Serves 4

100g (3½oz) rocket

½ lollo rosso lettuce, leaves ripped into strips

75g (2½oz) walnut pieces, toasted

50g (1¾oz) Parmesan shavings

Dressing

1 tablespoon apple cider vinegar

3 tablespoons extra virgin olive oil

salt and pepper

1 Place the rocket in a bowl with the lollo rosso leaves.

2 Whisk the dressing ingredients together and season.

3 Dress the salad leaves and sprinkle with the walnuts and Parmesan shavings.

Apple cider vinegar can help lower blood sugar levels and may even help to reduce cholesterol.

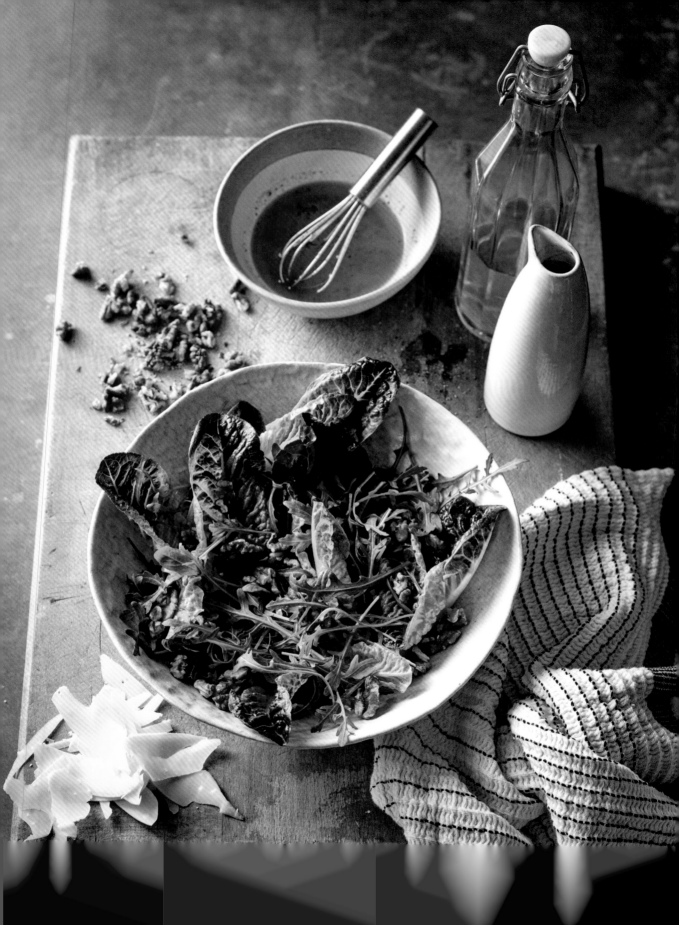

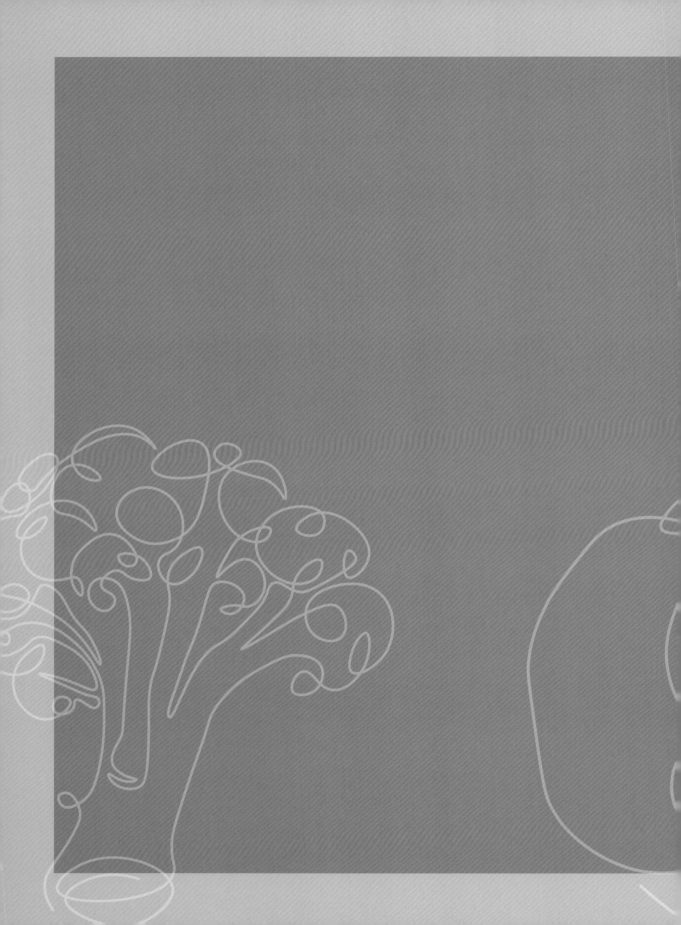

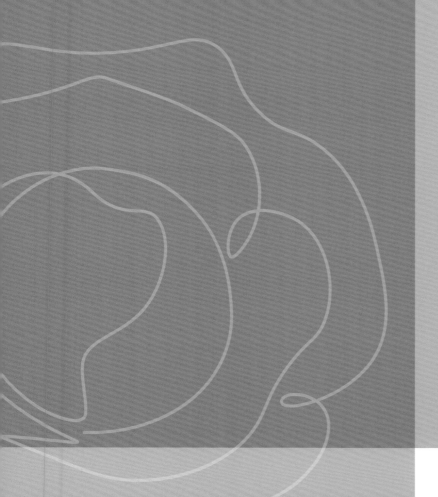

Veg

4

Braised chickpeas with celery, chard, carrots & tomato

A classic Italian chickpea dish that celebrates rainbow chard, stalks and all.

Serves 6

150g (5½oz) dried chickpeas, soaked overnight in lots of cold water

9 garlic cloves: 6 peeled and 3 crushed

1 red chilli

3 cherry tomatoes

1 sprig of rosemary

500g (1lb 2oz) rainbow chard

3 tablespoons olive oil

1 onion, finely chopped

300g (10½oz) carrots, peeled and cut into 1cm (½in) dice

4 celery sticks, cut into 1cm (½in) dice

pinch of chilli flakes

100ml (3½fl oz) white wine

75g (2½oz) passata

juice of 1 lemon

2 tablespoons chopped flat leaf parsley

extra virgin olive oil, for drizzling

salt and pepper

1 Drain the chickpeas and place in a saucepan with the peeled garlic, chilli, tomatoes and rosemary. Cover with cold water by a good 3cm (1¼in) and bring to the boil. Simmer for about 40 minutes or until the chickpeas are tender, adding more water if they seem to be dry. When cooked, season really well and set aside.

2 Prepare the rainbow chard by stripping the leaves from the stalks. Thinly slice the stalks and blanch the leaves in lots of boiling salted water for a minute. Drain and refresh in cold water. Squeeze out any excess moisture and roughly chop.

3 In a large pan, heat the olive oil and add the chopped onion, carrots, celery and chard stalks. Season and cook over a medium heat for about 15 minutes until the vegetables are just cooked without browning. Add the crushed garlic and chilli flakes and cook for another minute before pouring in the wine. Season well and reduce the wine to a syrup.

4 Drain the chickpeas, reserving the liquid, and add the pulses to the vegetables along with the passata. Simmer for 10 minutes, stirring well. Fold through the chard leaves with the lemon juice. Bring to a simmer, adding a little of the reserved chickpea cooking liquor if the mix is too dry. Stir through the chopped parsley and drizzle with good olive oil.

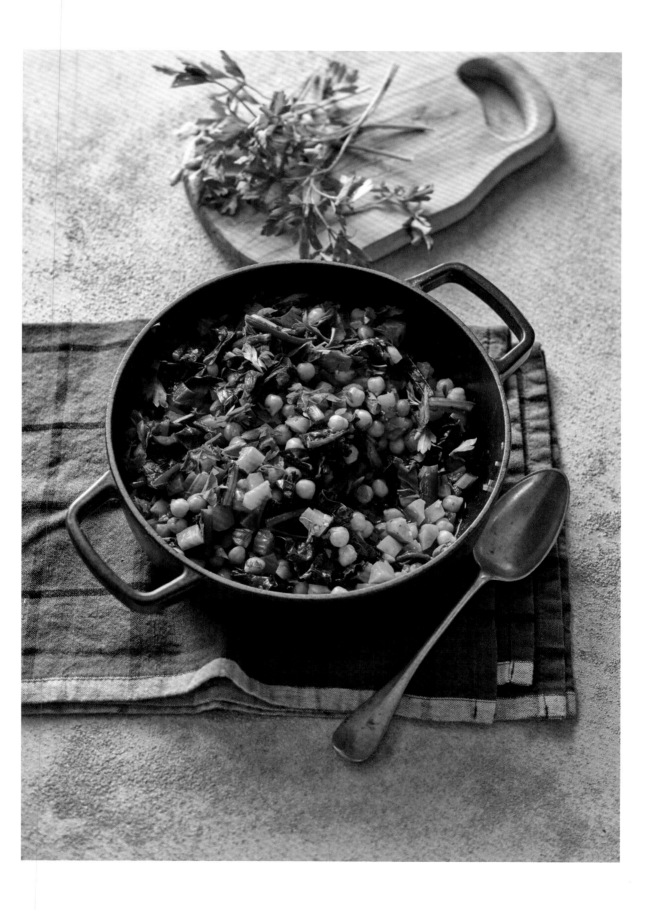

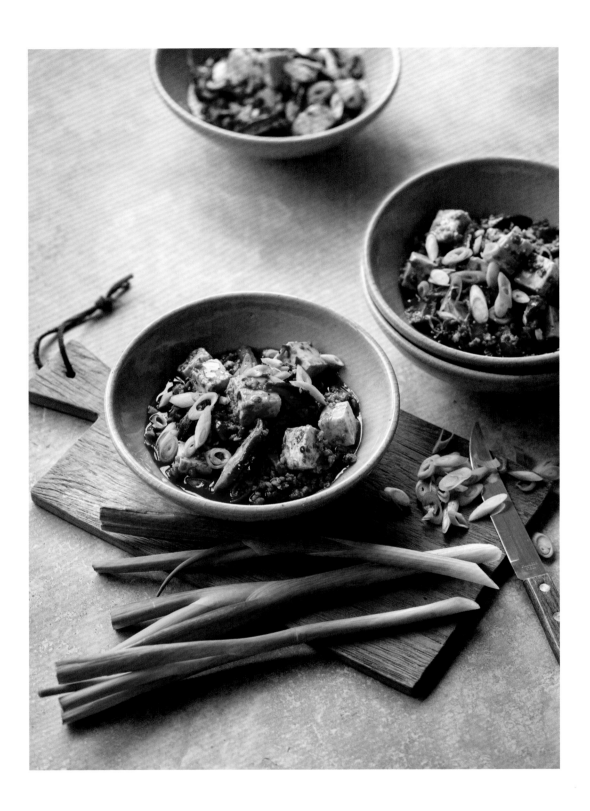

Mapo tofu

A vegan version of this classic Sichuan dish which usually contains minced pork.

Serves 4

2 tablespoons olive oil

2 teaspoons ground Sichuan pepper

pinch of chilli flakes

1 star anise

pinch of Chinese 5 spice

4 garlic cloves, crushed

3cm (1¼in) piece of fresh ginger, peeled and grated

200g (7oz) shiitake (or button) mushrooms, sliced

150g (5½oz) soy mince

2 tablespoons chilli bean paste (doubanjiang)

1 tablespoon light soy sauce

1 tablespoon rice wine or sherry

200ml (7fl oz) vegetable stock

400g (14oz) silken tofu

1 tablespoon sesame oil

1 bunch of spring onions, sliced

1 Heat the oil in a large, shallow pan. Add the spices with the garlic and ginger and stir over a low heat for 2 minutes. Add the sliced mushrooms with the soy mince, turn up the heat and stir-fry for a few minutes.

2 Reduce the heat and stir though the chilli bean paste, soy sauce, rice wine and vegetable stock. Simmer for 10 minutes or until you have a thick sauce.

3 Cut the tofu into 1–2cm (½–¾in) cubes and fold through the sauce. Simmer for 5 minutes to heat through and sprinkle with sesame oil.

4 Sprinkle with chopped spring onions to serve.

Garlic is an excellent source of manganese and vitamin B6 and, when eaten regularly, has anti-viral properties.

Braised red cabbage & radicchio with apple, blue cheese & pecans

A quick-cook red cabbage dish. Goat's cheese can be used instead of the blue, walnuts and hazelnuts instead of pecans.

Serves 4

2 tablespoons olive oil

1 red onion, thinly sliced

2 garlic cloves, crushed

2 tablespoons balsamic vinegar

⅙ red cabbage, cored and thinly shredded

1 head of radicchio, cored and shredded

2 apples, cored and cut into small pieces

75g (2½oz) toasted pecans, roughly chopped

100g (3½oz) blue cheese, cut into small pieces

2 tablespoons chopped flat leaf parsley

pinch of light soft brown sugar

salt and pepper

1 Heat the olive oil in a large pan and gently cook the red onion for a few minutes. Add the garlic and vinegar and turn up the heat. Tip in the red cabbage and stir well. Cook over a high heat, stirring constantly, until the red cabbage has wilted. Season well and add the radicchio. Cook for another 5 minutes.

2 Check the seasoning and stir through the apple, nuts, blue cheese and parsley. Add a little brown sugar and more vinegar if needed.

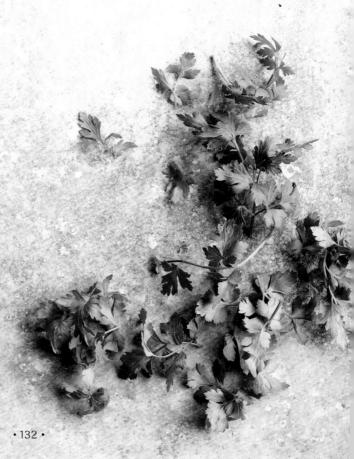

Beetroot & carrot poriyal

A classic southern Indian vegetable dish based on a recipe from a lovely lady who supplies me with curry leaves. The same method can be used with cabbage and lots of other shredded veg. Serve with a dhal or curry alongside Raita (page 176) and Kachumber (page 118) for a feast of vegetables and flavours.

Serves 4

2 tablespoons coconut oil

1 tablespoon black mustard seeds

15–20 fresh curry leaves

1 green chilli, deseeded and chopped

1 onion, finely chopped

½ teaspoon ground turmeric

1 teaspoon cumin seeds

3 tablespoons grated coconut

300g (10½oz) raw beetroot, peeled and grated

2 carrots, peeled and grated

juice of 1 lemon

salt and pepper

1 Heat the oil in a non-stick pan and add the mustard seeds, curry leaves and chilli. When the mustard seeds start to pop, add the onion, turmeric and cumin seeds and cook over a low heat for 5 minutes.

2 Add the coconut with the grated vegetables and stir-fry for a minute. Cover and cook over a low heat for 5 minutes until the vegetables have wilted and are just cooked. Add the lemon juice and season to taste.

The deep purple colour of beetroot comes from betalains, which have antioxidant and anti-inflammatory properties.

Fava bean purée with Padron peppers

Traditionally served with friggitelli peppers and braised chicory in Puglia, Padrons are used here as an alternative.

Serves 6

150g (5½oz) dried fava beans, soaked overnight in lots of cold water

12 garlic cloves: 10 peeled, 2 crushed

1 red chilli

3 cherry tomatoes

1 teaspoon fennel seeds, ground

½ teaspoon chilli flakes

2 garlic cloves, crushed

150ml (5fl oz) olive oil

200g (7oz) Padron peppers

salt and pepper

1   Drain the beans, place in a pan and cover with water. Add the garlic, chilli and tomatoes. Bring to the boil and simmer for about 20 minutes or until beans are tender. Season and remove from heat.

2   Drain the beans well and place in a food processor along with the fennel seeds, chilli flakes and crushed garlic. Pulse and steadily add 100ml (3½fl oz) of the olive oil until you have a smooth, thick purée.

3   In a frying pan over a medium heat, fry the Padron peppers in the remaining olive oil and sprinkle with salt. Keep stirring and remove from the heat when the peppers are slightly browned.

4   Serve the fava bean purée with Padrons.

★ Toasting vegetables

This method may be a little unorthodox, but it works well and emphasizes the flavour of the vegetables. Vegetables can be placed directly between the plates of a sandwich toaster or panini-style grill. They tend to char slightly and steam at the same time. The results are so good. The obvious one to start with is asparagus but broccoli, cauliflower, leeks, French beans, runner beans, pak choi and cabbage cook well using this method. Even kale can be cooked this way!

Having an olive oil and vinegar dressing ready is a great idea (see rocket salad dressing page 124) and as the vegetables cook, they can be tossed in the dressing while still warm.

Squash, corn & bean cakes

The mixed seed coating provides some crunch to the cakes, and great flavour.

Serves 6

2 tablespoons olive oil, plus extra for frying the cakes

1 onion, chopped

1 teaspoon paprika

½ teaspoon ground turmeric

pinch of ground cumin

1 garlic clove, crushed

100g (3½oz) red piquillo peppers or peeled peppers, chopped

2 tablespoons passata

cooked corn from 2 cobs (or 200g canned sweetcorn, drained)

100g (3½oz) cannellini beans (canned or cooked from dried beans

100g (3½oz) kidney beans (canned or cooked from dry beans)

500g (1lb 2oz) diced roasted squash or pumpkin

juice of ½ lime

salt and pepper

Coating

gram flour

2 eggs, beaten

100g (3½oz) Seed mix (page 181), roughly chopped

1 Cook the onion in the oil with the paprika, turmeric and cumin. Stir in the garlic and red pepper and cook for another minute. Add the passata and corn kernels and simmer for 5 minutes.

2 Roughly mash half of the beans and stir into the mix with the roasted squash. Season well and add the lime juice. Mix well and leave to cool.

3 Shape into small patties and refrigerate for about 45 minutes.

4 Turn each bean cake firstly in the gram flour, then the beaten egg and finally the seeds. Heat 3 tablespoons of olive oil in a non- stick frying pan and fry the cakes for a few minutes on each side until golden brown and crisp.

5 Serve with an avocado and tomato salsa or Kimchi miso mayonnaise (page 185).

Cooking sweetcorn makes its antioxidants easier to absorb.

Cap chay

This Indonesian dish uses dried bean curd sheets as well as lots of vegetables to make a substantial meal. Bean curd sheets can be used as an alternative to pasta or dumpling wrappers.

Serves 6

15g (½oz) dried wood ear mushrooms

75g (2½oz) dried bean curd sheets

3 tablespoons olive oil

3 garlic cloves, crushed

3cm (1¼in) piece of fresh ginger, peeled and grated

150g (5½oz) shiitake mushrooms, sliced

3 carrots, peeled and cut into batons

500g (1lb 2oz) Chinese cabbage, thinly sliced

1 tablespoon fermented bean curd paste (taucheo)

3 tablespoons light soy sauce

1 tablespoon oyster sauce (or vegetarian alternative)

1 tablespoon sesame oil

2 teaspoons honey

100g (3½oz) sugar snap peas, sliced

100g (3½oz) beansprouts

2 tablespoons chopped chives

1 Soak the wood ear mushrooms in plenty of just boiled water for at least 20 minutes, then drain and slice. Soak the bean curd sheets in hot water for 15 minutes and cut into 4cm (1½in) pieces.

2 In a large wok, heat the oil, add the garlic, ginger, mushrooms, bean curd sheets, carrots and cabbage. Stir-fry for a few minutes over a high heat, then add the bean curd paste, soy and oyster sauces, sesame oil and honey. Stir to combine and bring to a simmer. Cover and simmer for about 15 minutes.

3 Add the sugar snaps, beansprouts and chives. Taste for seasoning and add more soy or honey if required. Cover and leave for another 5 minutes before serving.

When mushrooms are exposed to sunlight (UV), it increases their concentration of vitamin D. Try putting them on the windowsill for a couple of hours at midday for a dose of natural vitamin D.

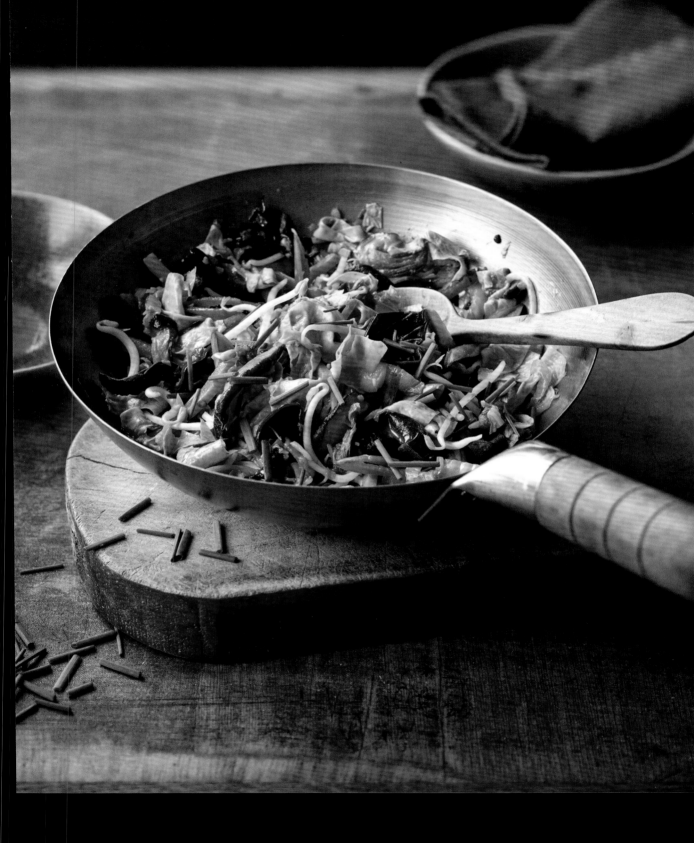

Miso-glazed aubergines

**The toppings give texture to this Japanese dish.
Serve with braised spinach or other greens.**

Serves 4

4 aubergines

2 tablespoons olive oil

Glaze

4 tablespoons white miso paste

2 tablespoons sake

2 tablespoons mirin

1 tablespoon light soy sauce

1 tablespoon maple syrup

2 teaspoons finely grated fresh ginger

Toppings

2 tablespoons chopped pickled ginger

6 spring onions, chopped

1 tablespoon sesame seeds

1 tablespoon black sesame seeds

2 tablespoons puffed barley

2 tablespoons sev

1 Preheat the oven to 180°C (350°F/gas mark 4).

2 Cut each aubergine in half lengthways and score the cut sides in squares by making diagonal cuts. The cuts should be about 5mm–1cm (¼–½in) deep without cutting through into the skin.

3 Heat the oil in a large non-stick pan and place the aubergines cut-side down in the oil. Fry for 3–4 minutes over a medium heat to brown, flip over and do the same on the skin side. This may have to be done in batches. Place the aubergines flesh-side up on a baking tray.

4 Mix the glaze ingredients together in a pan and whisk together over a low heat until the sauce is smooth and thick. Brush the miso glaze over the aubergines, coating well. Reserve any remaining for serving. Bake in the oven for 15–20 minutes or until the aubergines are tender.

5 Serve drizzled with extra glaze and sprinkled with the topping ingredients.

Aubergine polpettine

A perfect alternative to meatballs, with a good basic tomato sauce that can also be used with pasta.

Serves 4

2 large aubergines, peeled

2 tablespoons olive oil

1 garlic clove, crushed

½ teaspoon dried oregano

1 egg, beaten

2 tablespoons chopped basil

1 tablespoon chopped flat leaf parsley

1 tablespoon chopped mint

1 tablespoon capers (salted or in vinegar), soaked in plenty of cold water for 15 minutes and rinsed

100g (3½oz) ground almonds

50g (1¾oz) grated Parmesan

gram flour, for coating

olive oil, for frying

salt and pepper

Tomato sauce

2 tablespoons olive oil

10 garlic cloves, thinly sliced

2 red chillies, deseeded and chopped

600g (1lb 5oz) canned chopped tomatoes

pinch of sugar

To serve

10 black olives, roughly chopped

fresh basil leaves

grated Parmesan

1 To make the tomato sauce, warm the oil in a pan and cook the garlic and chillies for a few minutes until the garlic is opaque but not browning. Add the tomatoes and sugar and bring to a simmer. Cook over a low heat for about 30 minutes until you have a reduced and thick sauce. Season well and blend until smooth.

2 Slice the peeled aubergines into rounds of 5mm–1cm (¼–½ in) thick. Cut each slice into small dice. Heat the oil in a non-stick frying pan. Add the aubergine dice and fry over a high heat to lightly brown. Add the garlic and oregano, stir through and cover the pan. Turn the heat down and allow the veg to steam for about 10 minutes until soft. Season well.

3 When cool, add the egg, herbs, capers, almonds and cheese. Mix well and add seasoning. Shape into small balls and roll in gram flour to coat. Wipe out the non-stick pan. Add a few tablespoons of olive oil and fry the balls until lightly browned. Tip in the tomato sauce and simmer for about 10 minutes.

4 Top with the chopped olives, basil and Parmesan to serve.

Fish

5

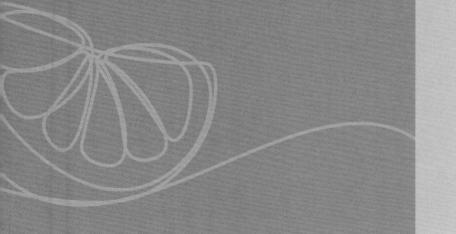

Sesame coconut fish with braised spinach

Chard, kale or other greens can be used instead of spinach, but blanch them first in boiling water before braising. Any white fish can be used for this recipe, but the firmer the better. The flavours are good with salmon fillets too.

Serves 4

4 x 150g (5½oz) fillets of skinless white fish, such as sea bass

2 tablespoons coconut oil

300g (10½oz) spinach

1 tablespoon olive oil

2 teaspoons grated fresh ginger

½ teaspoon chilli flakes

lime wedges to serve

Paste

1 teaspoon maple syrup

2 teaspoons oyster sauce

1 egg, beaten

2 tablespoons sesame seeds

2 tablespoons desiccated coconut

1 garlic clove, crushed

1 tablespoon chopped coriander

½ teaspoon ground turmeric

1 In a bowl, mix together all the paste ingredients to make a stiff paste. Spread the paste over the fish fillets and place in the fridge for at least 1 hour for the paste to become firm.

2 Preheat the oven to 160°C (325°F/gas mark 3).

3 In a large, non-stick, ovenproof frying pan, heat the coconut oil and place the fish fillets paste-side down. Cook for a few minutes until the paste is nicely browned, then flip over the fish carefully using a spatula, trying not to break the crust. Place the pan in the oven for 7–8 minutes or until the fish is cooked. Remove from the oven and leave to rest for a few minutes.

4 Meanwhile, wash the spinach and drain well. Heat the oil in a large pan. Add the ginger and chilli flakes and cook for a minute before adding the spinach. Stir very well and wilt the spinach in the pan over a high heat. Tip the greens into a colander over a bowl to drain out any excess moisture.

5 Place the fish on top of the spinach and add lime wedges to serve.

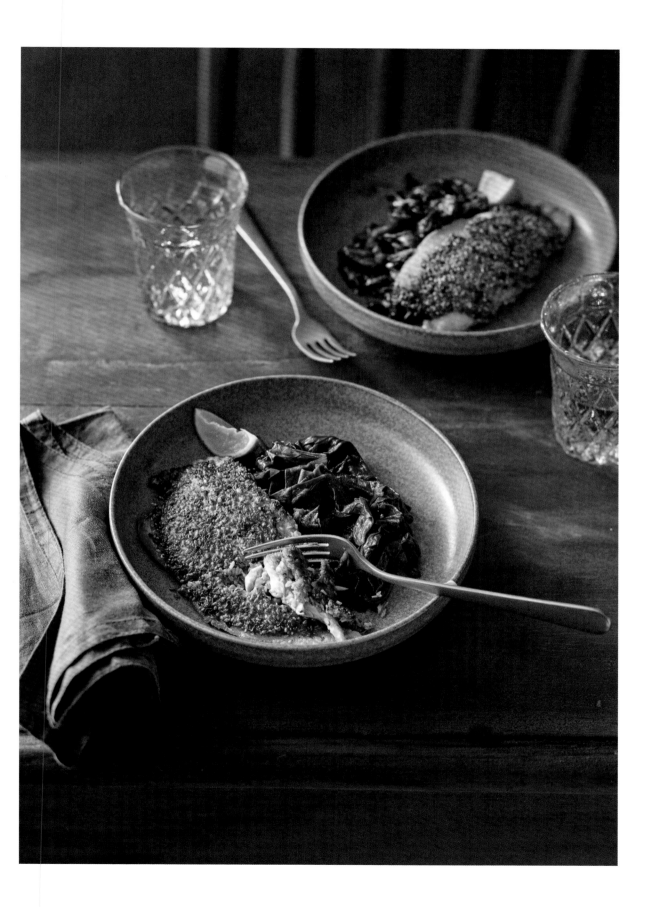

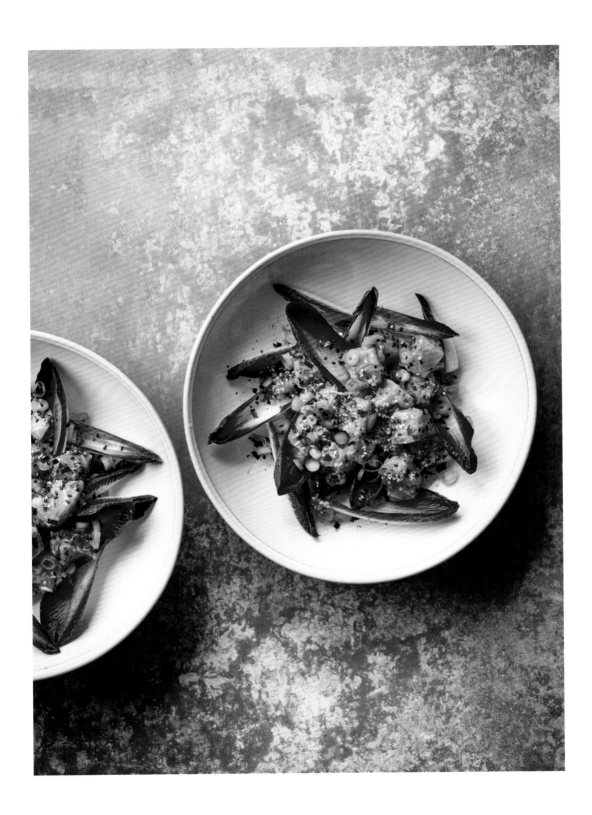

Salmon poke

This Hawaiian dish is traditionally made with very-good-quality tuna, so please use it if you have access to it, but it's also great with other oily fish, like mackerel. You can make this into a more substantial meal by adding the following, along with some cooked grains like buckwheat or barley: Pickled cucumber (page 176), spicy slaw (page 120), Kimchi miso mayonnaise (page 185).

Serves 4

500g (1lb 2oz) salmon fillet

2 teaspoons sesame oil

1 tablespoon rice wine vinegar

juice of ½ lime

3 tablespoons tamari or light soy sauce

2 red chillies, deseeded and chopped

3cm (1¼in) piece of fresh ginger, peeled and finely grated

1 bunch of spring onions, chopped

2 tablespoons sesame seeds, toasted

3 heads of red chicory

1 tablespoon black sesame seeds

good sprinkle of furikake

1. Skin the salmon and cut into 1cm (½in) cubes.

2. Mix the sesame oil with the vinegar, lime juice, tamari, chilli, ginger, spring onions and sesame seeds. Whisk well to combine and add the fish to the mix.

3. While the fish is marinating, separate the leaves from the red chicory and arrange on a serving plate. Spoon the fish onto the leaves and sprinkle with black sesame seeds and furikake to serve.

As well as being rich in omega-3 fatty acids, salmon is a good source of protein, B vitamins, potassium and selenium. It is also lower in mercury and rich in iron.

Seared tuna & soba noodle salad

This dish benefits from the addition of the Pickled cucumber on page 176. Other vegetables can be used in the noodle salad.

Serves 4

2 tablespoons tamari or light soy sauce

1 tablespoon sesame oil

1 tablespoon honey

1 tablespoon rice vinegar

4 x 100g (3½oz) good-quality tuna steaks

150g (5½oz) soba noodles

100g (3½oz) cooked edamame

6 spring onions, chopped

1 red pepper, deseeded and thinly sliced

1 carrot, peeled and grated

1/6 red cabbage, thinly sliced

8 cherry tomatoes, halved

2 tablespoons roughly chopped coriander

3 tablespoons olive oil

2 tablespoons white and black sesame seeds

lime wedges, to serve

Dressing

2 tablespoons rice vinegar

2 teaspoons grated ginger

1 garlic clove, crushed

juice of ½ lime

2 teaspoons sriracha

2 tablespoons sesame oil

2 tablespoons tamari or light soy sauce

2 teaspoons white miso paste

1   Mix the tamari, sesame oil, honey and rice vinegar together. Turn the tuna steaks in the marinade and leave for about 1 hour.

2   Cook the soba noodles in lots of salted water as per the packet instructions. Drain and refresh with lots of running cold water. Toss with the vegetables, tomatoes and coriander.

3   Whisk together all the dressing ingredients and fold through the salad.

4   Heat the oil in a non-stick frying pan. Take the tuna out of its marinade and coat in the sesame seeds. Cook for 1–2 minutes on each side, depending on the thickness. The tuna should be rare in the middle.

5   Serve with the noodle salad and wedges of lime.

Miso is high in salt but is also protein- and nutrient-rich and is a fermented food, great for our gut microbiome.

Smoked fish with beetroot, orange, caraway & horseradish

Beetroot flavoured with caraway and orange is a great favourite. Quinoa pancakes (page 96) could be served alongside this dish.

Serves 4

300g (10½oz) raw beetroot, peeled and cut into batons 1cm (½in) thick

2 tablespoons olive oil

1 tablespoon balsamic vinegar

1 tablespoon maple syrup

150g (5½oz) Greek yogurt

1 shallot, chopped

1 tablespoon chopped chives, plus extra to garnish

1 tablespoon creamed horseradish

60g (2¼oz) wild rocket

¼ head of radicchio, shredded

150g (5½oz) cooked Puy lentils

200g (7oz) smoked salmon, eel or other smoked fish (or plain cooked salmon)

salt and pepper

Dressing

1 tablespoon olive oil

2 teaspoons caraway seeds

1 garlic clove, crushed

zest and juice of 1 large orange

1 teaspoon honey

1 tablespoon balsamic vinegar

1 Preheat the oven to 160°C (325°F/gas mark 3).

2 Toss the beetroot in a baking tray with the oil, vinegar and maple syrup. Season well and cover tightly with foil. Bake for about 30-40 minutes or until the beetroot is tender. When cooked, check the seasoning again and set aside.

3 To make the dressing, heat the olive oil in a small pan. Tip in the caraway seeds with the garlic and cook for a minute without browning the garlic. Quickly add the orange zest and juice along with the honey and balsamic vinegar and reduce to a thin syrup. While still hot, toss the syrup through the beetroot.

4 Mix the yogurt with the shallot, chives and horseradish. Season well.

5 In a large bowl, toss the salad leaves with the lentils. Fold through the beetroot with all of the juices and transfer to a serving plate. Dollop the yogurt over the salad and drape pieces of the fish over the dish. Finish with a sprinkling of chives.

Sicilian sardine pasta

A great way to enjoy pasta with plenty of fibre, protein, healthy fats and flavour. Fresh sardines can be used but the canned fish make a quick, cheap and authentic alternative.

Serves 4

2 tablespoons sultanas

1 red onion, finely chopped

½ head of fennel, finely chopped

pinch of saffron strands (optional)

1 teaspoon chilli flakes

1 teaspoon ground fennel seeds

2 tablespoons olive oil

2 garlic cloves, crushed

6 anchovy fillets

2 x 120g (4¼oz) cans sardines in olive oil

3 tablespoons white wine

400g (14oz) spelt linguine or spaghetti

2 tablespoons pine nuts (or flaked almonds), toasted

2 tablespoons chopped flat leaf parsley

good olive oil, for drizzling

salt and pepper

1 In a small bowl, cover the sultanas with boiling water and set aside.

2 In a large, shallow pan, cook the red onion, fennel, saffron (if using), chilli flakes and fennel seeds in the olive oil over a medium heat for 10 minutes without colouring the onion. Add the garlic and cook gently for another 5 minutes. Tip in the anchovy fillets and remove the pan from the heat. Stir well until the anchovies have dissolved into the onion mixture.

3 Drain the canned sardines and cut each one into 3 pieces. Add to the pan with the wine. Return to the heat for a few minutes, stirring to combine, until heated through.

4 Cook the pasta in lots of boiling salted water as per the packet instructions. Drain and return to the pan along with the warm sardine sauce.

5 Drain the sultanas and add them to the pasta with the nuts and parsley. Mix well and season.

6 Serve drizzled with some good olive oil.

 Other pasta sauce ideas

There is a traditional northern Italian pasta dish called pizzoccheri using buckwheat pasta strips. The sauce consists of cabbage, potatoes, fontina cheese and butter, which is a little heavy. However, a sauce with sautéed cabbage, walnuts, blue cheese, roast cauliflower and Parmesan would make a healthier option to use with the buckwheat pasta.

· **Kale and nut pesto** (page 186)

· **The tomato sauce from Aubergine polpettine** (page 139).

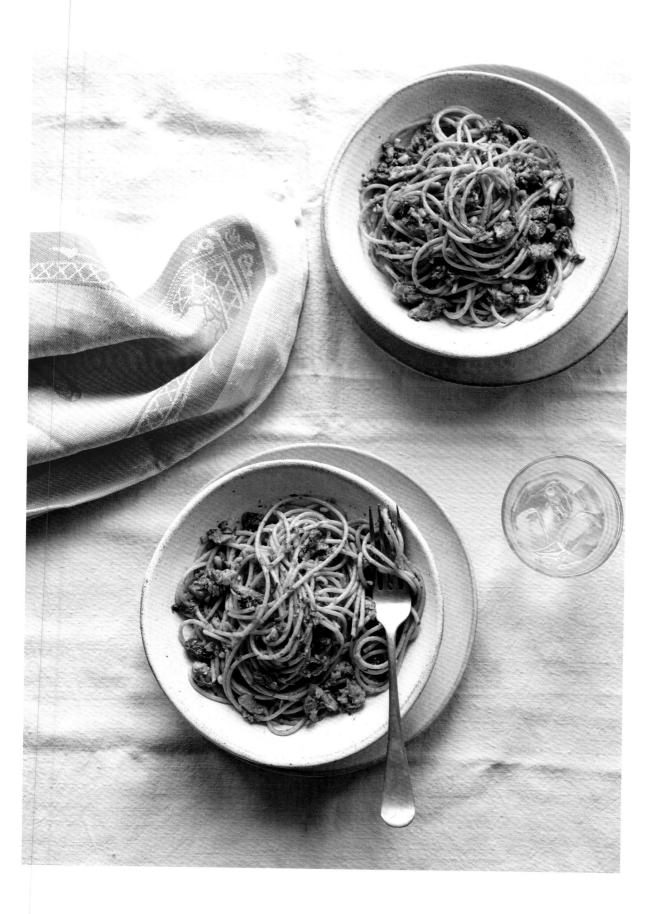

Salmon with fennel, olives & tomatoes

A very quick dish to make that is lovely at room temperature. It brings together vegetables, beans, omega-3-rich fish and polyphenol-rich herbs for a delicious and nutritious option. The salad can also be used as a side for other fish dishes.

Serves 4

3 tablespoons olive oil

4 x 125g (4½oz) salmon pieces, skin removed

20 cherry tomatoes

4 anchovy fillets, chopped

12 black olives

2 tablespoons balsamic vinegar

salt and pepper

Salad

100g (3½oz) cannellini beans (canned or cooked from dried)

1 head of fennel, finely sliced

1 red onion, finely sliced

100g (3½oz) French beans, blanched

1 garlic clove, crushed

1 tablespoon chopped flat leaf parsley

3 tablespoons olive oil

1 Preheat the oven to 180°C (350°F/gas mark 4).

2 Rinse the cannellini beans and put in a bowl with the remaining salad ingredients. Fold together to combine and set aside. Season to taste.

3 Heat the olive oil in a shallow, ovenproof frying pan and fry the salmon pieces on all sides, seasoning well. Add the tomatoes, anchovy fillets and olives. Cover and place the pan in a the oven for about 5 minutes or until the salmon is just cooked.

4 Place the salad on a serving dish and top with the salmon and all the pan contents. Drizzle with balsamic vinegar.

Mackerel escabeche

Salmon or trout can be used instead of the mackerel, along with other oily fish. Using a variety of colourful herbs and spices, this dish serves up plenty of polyphenols.

Serves 4

1 red onion, thinly sliced

2 garlic cloves, crushed

1 green chilli, deseeded and sliced

½ red pepper, deseeded and sliced

½ head of fennel, thinly sliced

1 small carrot, peeled and cut into thin slices on the diagonal

zest and juice of 1 orange

1 bay leaf

1 sprig of thyme

1 tablespoon maple syrup

50ml (2fl oz) moscatel vinegar

2 tablespoons gram flour

2 teaspoons smoked paprika

6 mackerel fillets

50ml (2fl oz) olive oil

good-quality extra virgin olive oil, for drizzling

salt and pepper

1 Place all the ingredients up to and including the vinegar in a pan and bring to the boil. Simmer for 10 minutes until the vegetables are just tender. Check the balance between sweet and sour, adding more vinegar or syrup as required.

2 Mix the gram flour with the smoked paprika and seasoning and place in a shallow bowl. Cut the mackerel fillets into 3cm (1¼in) pieces and toss in the flour until well coated.

3 In a non-stick frying pan, heat the oil and fry the mackerel pieces for a minute on each side, in batches if necessary. Remove the fish to a serving dish. When all the mackerel is part-cooked, tip over the pickling mix and drizzle with extra virgin olive oil. Turn the fish pieces over in the mix and leave for at least 1 hour for the flavours to improve.

An oily fish rich in omega-3s, mackerel is a good source of protein and B vitamins, particularly vitamin B12 and is very low mercury as well as being a more sustainable fish to enjoy regularly.

Sea bass, radicchio, lentil & porcini parcels

A delicious dish with a variety of brilliant plants, including mushrooms, lentils and fresh parsley. These bags can be put together ahead of time and cooked just before serving.

Serves 4

4 x 150g (5½oz) fillets of sea bass, skin on and descaled

20g (¾oz) dried porcini

150ml (5fl oz) boiling water

25g (1oz) salted butter

150g (5½oz) chestnut mushrooms, sliced

1 garlic clove, crushed

1 tablespoon chopped flat leaf parsley

2 tablespoons olive oil

½ head of radicchio, sliced

150g (5½oz) cooked Puy lentils

4 sprigs of thyme

100ml (3½fl oz) white wine

salt and pepper

1 Season the fish fillets well with salt and leave in the fridge until needed.

2 Soak the dried porcini in the boiling water for at least 20 minutes.

3 In a small frying pan, heat the butter until just melted, then tip in the mushrooms with the garlic and sauté over a high heat for a few minutes. Tip in the soaked porcini with their soaking liquor and reduce with the mushrooms until it is a syrupy consistency. Season well, stir through the parsley and remove from the heat to cool.

4 Preheat the oven to 180°C (350°F/gas mark 4).

5 Cut 4 large pieces of baking parchment big enough to fold over and make a large parcel containing the fish. Brush each one with olive oil and layer up each with a quarter of the radicchio, lentils and mushrooms, seasoning each layer. Place a fillet of bass on top (skin-side down) and top with a sprig of thyme. Drizzle with a little olive oil and one-quarter of the white wine each. Fold the parchment over and fold the open sides in to seal. I find that a stapler can help with the seal.

6 Place the parcels on a baking tray and cook for 15 minutes. Remove from the oven and leave to rest for 5 minutes before opening the bags carefully and sliding the contents gently onto plates.

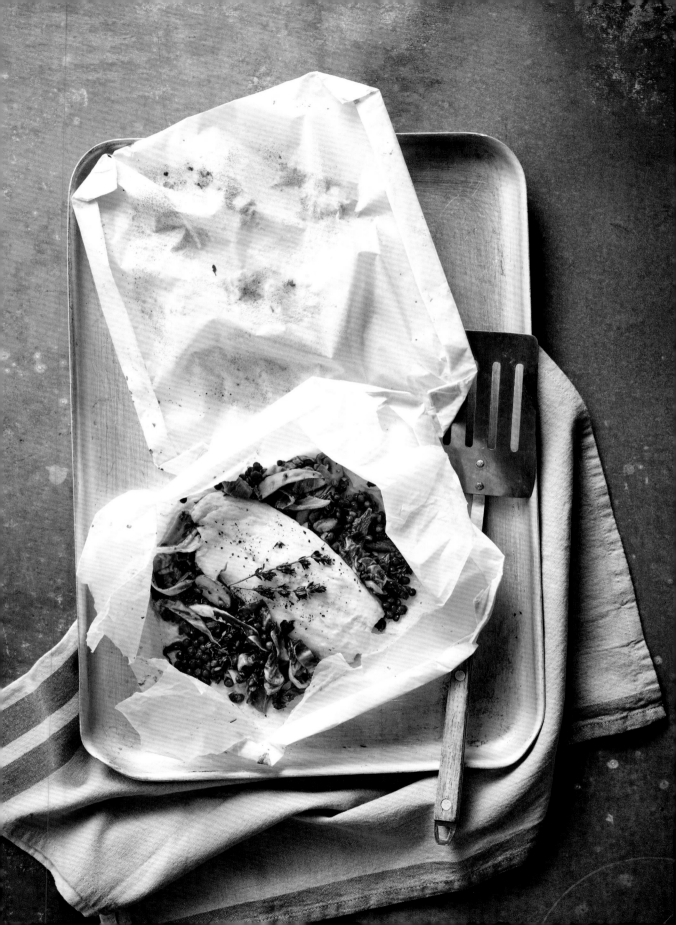

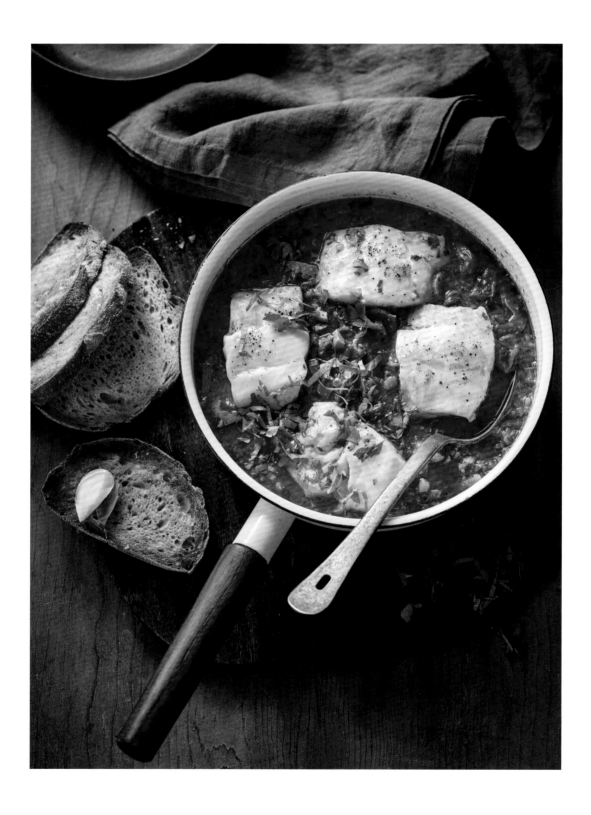

Pesce all'acqua pazza or poached fish in 'crazy water'

Most white fish can be used in this recipe – hake, cod, sea bass, for example. Traditionally, water is used in the recipe, but I prefer to use fish stock as it adds more flavour. More chilli can be added if you prefer more heat. This is usually served with toasted bread, rubbed with garlic.

Serves 4

3 tablespoons olive oil

1 small red onion, chopped

1 head of fennel, thinly sliced

4 garlic cloves, crushed

1 red chilli, deseeded and chopped

2 teaspoons ground fennel seeds

4 anchovy fillets

2 tablespoons capers (salted or in vinegar), rinsed

300g (10½oz) yellow and red cherry tomatoes, halved

120ml (4fl oz) white wine

500ml (18fl oz) fish stock or water

small bunch of basil, leaves shredded

1 tablespoon chopped flat leaf parsley

6 black olives, roughly chopped

4 x 150g (5½oz) white fish fillets, skin on and descaled

good-quality extra virgin olive oil, for drizzling

salt and pepper

1 Heat the oil in a large, shallow pan and add the onion and fennel. Cook over a medium heat for about 10 minutes without colouring. Add the garlic, chilli and fennel seeds and cook for a few more minutes over a low heat, stirring well. Add the anchovies and capers, take off the heat and beat until the anchovies have dissolved into the mixture.

2 Tip in the cherry tomatoes and return to a medium heat, then cook the tomatoes for about 5 minutes. Tip in the white wine and simmer for 5 minutes to reduce. Add the fish stock along with the herbs and olives. Simmer for about 15 minutes or until the liquid has reduced by about half.

3 Sprinkle the fish with salt. Place the fish on top of the tomato base, skin-side down, and bring back up to a simmer. Cover the pan and simmer gently for about 5 minutes or until the fish is firm to touch.

4 Drizzle the dish with extra virgin olive oil to serve.

Miso cod with braised greens

This recipe has to be started 2 days in advance as the fish will need at least 24 hours to marinate. Sea bass, hake or salmon are good substitutes.

Serves 4

75ml (2½fl oz) sake

75ml (2½fl oz) mirin

100g (3½oz) white miso paste

1 tablespoon honey

4 x 150g (5½oz) cod fillets, skin on and descaled

2 teaspoons grated fresh ginger

1 red chilli, deseeded and chopped

1 garlic clove, crushed

2 tablespoons olive oil

250g (9oz) pak choi, trimmed and quartered lengthways

125g (4½oz) asparagus, trimmed

125g (4½oz) French beans, trimmed

1 tablespoon sesame seeds, toasted

1 tablespoon black sesame seeds

1 tablespoon chopped chives

salt and pepper

1 Two days before cooking, make the marinade. In a small pan, simmer the sake and mirin together over a high heat for about 30 seconds. Add the miso and whisk into the mix over a very low heat until it has dissolved. Stir in the honey. Leave to cool to room temperature.

2 Pour two-thirds of the marinade over the cod in a shallow tray. Turn the cod over so it is well coated. Cover and place in the fridge for at least 24 hours and up to 2 days. Reserve the rest of the marinade.

3 In a large pan, cook the ginger, chilli and garlic in 1 tablespoon of the olive oil for a few minutes without colouring the garlic. Turn off the heat.

4 In a large pan of boiling salted water, cook the vegetables for a few minutes until just cooked. Drain well and transfer to the pan with the ginger and garlic mixture. Toss the vegetables and toasted sesame seeds in the mixture and season.

5 Preheat the oven to 200°C (400°F/gas mark 6).

6 Remove the fish from the marinade and wipe off any excess. Heat the remaining tablespoon of oil in a non-stick, ovenproof frying pan. Place the cod in the pan flesh-side down and cook for 2 minutes until lightly browned. Carefully flip the fish over and cook for another 2 minutes before transferring to the oven for 5–7 minutes until the cod is just cooked. The time will depend on the thickness of the cod and the appearance will be opaque, but it will be ready when just flaking apart. Alternatively, the fish can be cooked by placing on a tray under a grill or salamander.

7 Gently heat the remaining marinade. To serve, arrange the cod with the vegetables, drizzle with the marinade and sprinkle with black sesame seeds and chopped chives.

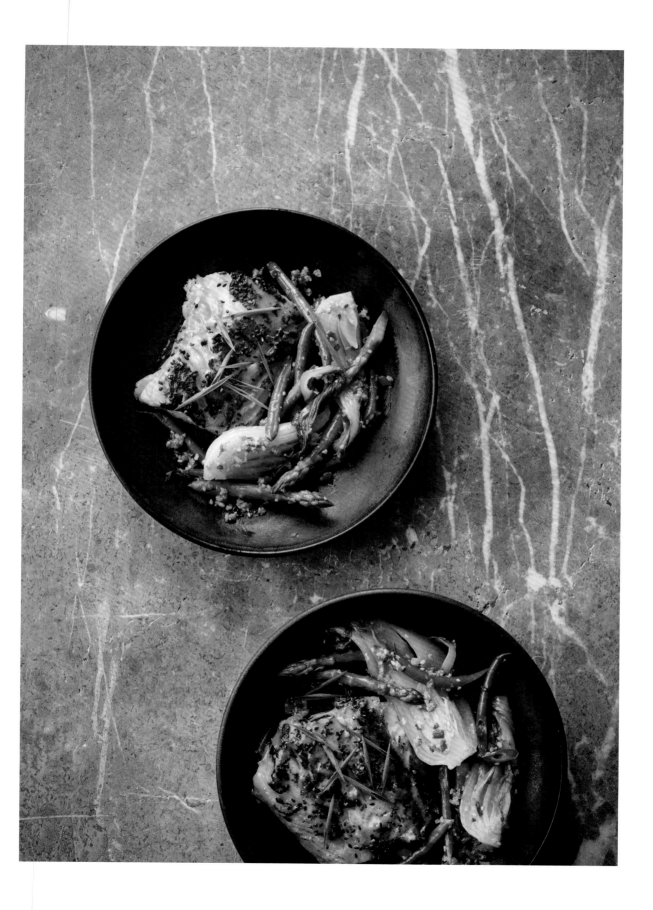

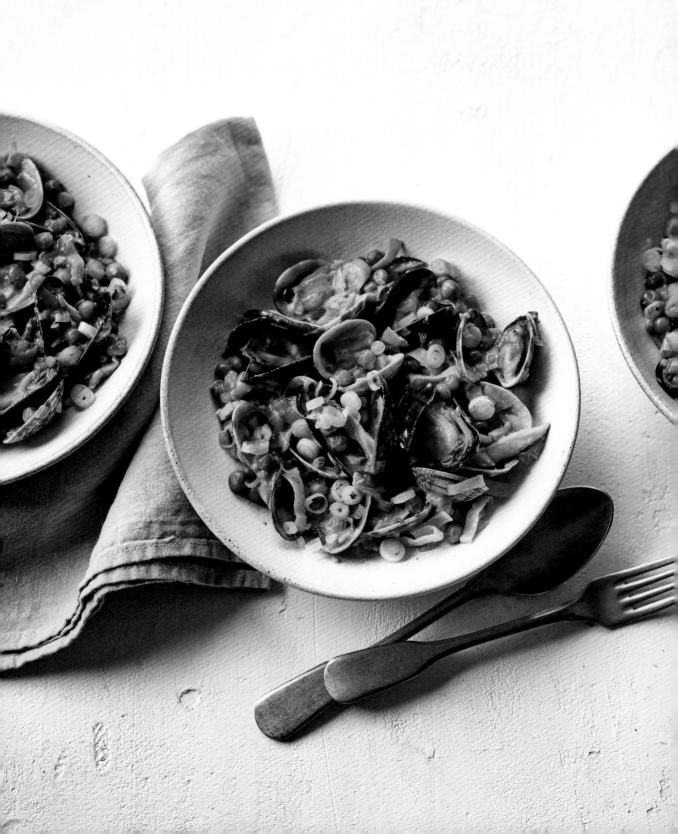

Mussels & clams with leeks, peas & shiitake mushrooms

Shellfish are the unsung heroes of seafood. More sustainable than most fish and rich in nutrients, they make a delicious meal. It's important the shellfish are just opened before they are removed from the pan, as they will continue to steam on standing. The combination of the miso and the reduced shellfish liquor makes a lovely sauce.

Serves 4

2 tablespoons olive oil

2 shallots, finely chopped

2 garlic cloves, crushed

1 tablespoon grated fresh ginger

2 leeks, finely sliced

100g (3½oz) shiitake mushrooms, sliced

200ml (7fl oz) sake (or sherry)

400g (14oz) fresh mussels, cleaned

400g (14oz) fresh clams

150g (5½oz) frozen peas

2 tablespoons white miso paste

6 spring onions, sliced

1 In a large pan, heat the oil with the shallots, garlic and ginger. Cook gently for 5 minutes, then tip in the leeks and shiitake. Cook for 5 minutes until just tender. Pour in the sake and bring to a simmer.

2 Tip in the mussels and clams and stir quickly. Turn up the heat and cover. Cook over a very high heat for about 3 minutes or until the shellfish have just opened. Using a slotted spoon remove the shellfish to a serving dish, discarding any that remain closed, then add the peas.

3 Reduce the remaining liquid until it is the consistency of single cream. Remove from the heat and whisk in the miso paste.

4 To serve, pour the pea sauce over the shellfish and sprinkle with the chopped spring onions.

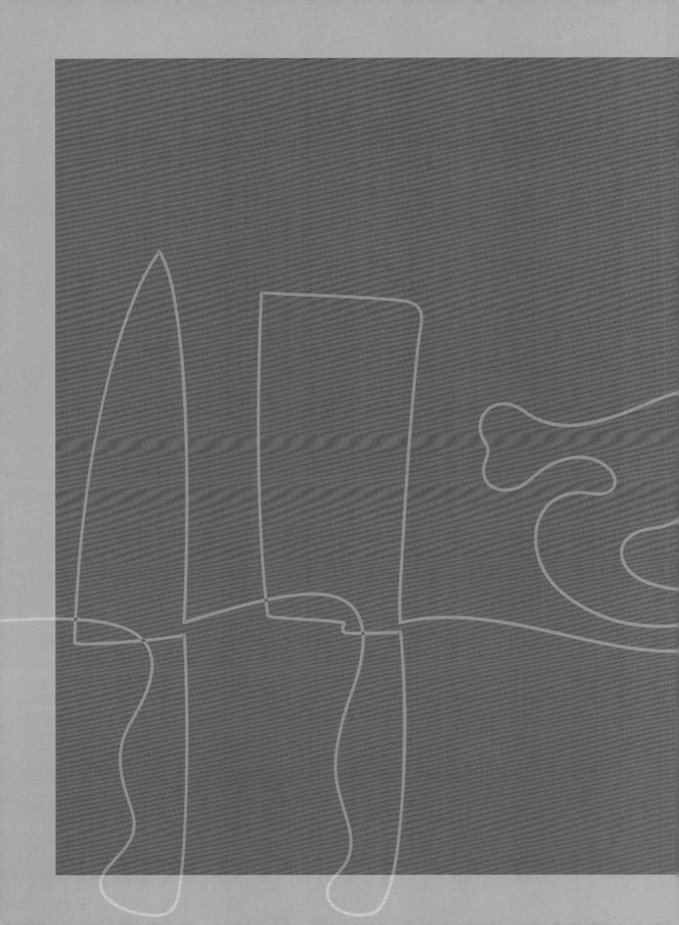

Meat

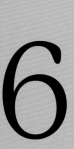

Baked kefir chicken

The kefir tenderizes the chicken and gives a wonderful flavour with the fresh herbs. Serve with a dressed green salad or mixed vegetables.

Serves 4

8 skinless, bone-in chicken
  thighs

300ml (10fl oz) kefir

2 garlic cloves, crushed

zest of 1 lemon

2 tablespoons chopped
  tarragon

2 tablespoons chopped flat
  leaf parsley

2 tablespoons chopped chives

salt and pepper

1 Slice each chicken thigh across the bone a few times and place in a shallow container. In a food processor, blend the rest of the ingredients together and pour over the chicken, turning it in the marinade until well coated. Cover and leave in the fridge to marinate overnight.

2 Take the chicken out of the fridge 30 minutes before cooking to allow it to come up to room temperature.

3 Preheat the oven to 180°C (350°F/gas mark 4).

4 Place the chicken in a shallow baking tray with all of the marinade and juices and cook for about 30 minutes or until the juices run clear.

Chicken is a lean source of protein and the darker leg meat is rich in minerals such as iron, selenium and zinc. Buy high welfare, organic chicken where possible.

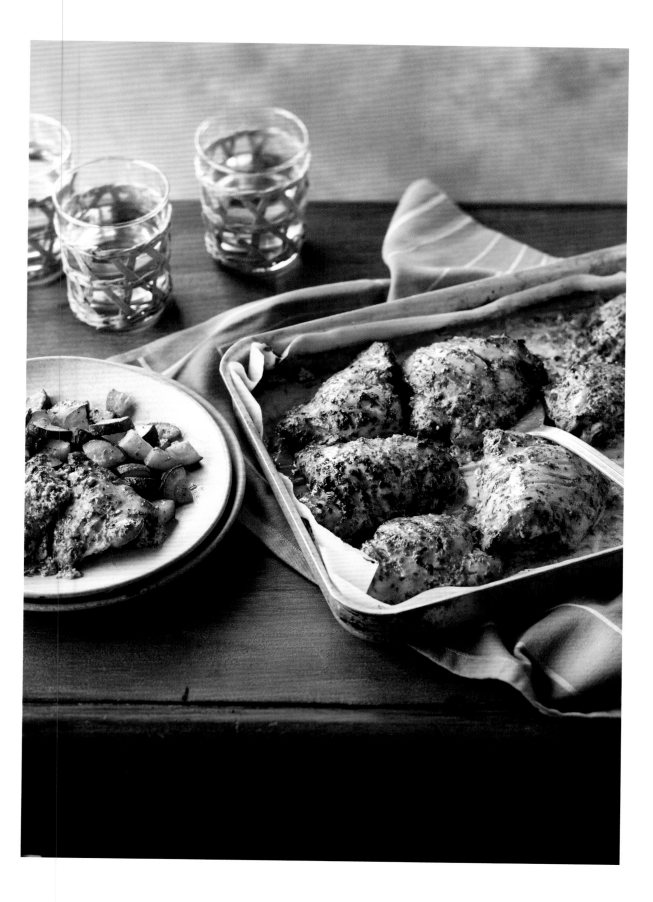

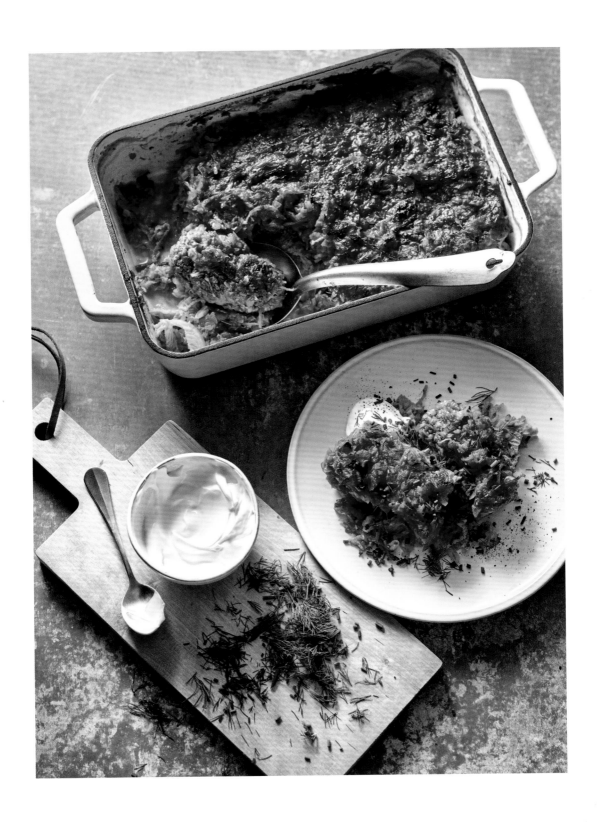

Baked cabbage rolls

Cabbages are often neglected and underused. This dish makes the most of them in both their fresh and fermented forms. Fibre and probiotics in one delicious dish.

Serves 4-6

1 Savoy cabbage

400g (14oz) sauerkraut

500g (1lb 2oz) minced turkey

200g (7oz) ricotta

1 egg, beaten

3 tablespoons olive oil

2 onions, finely chopped

4 garlic cloves, crushed

1 tablespoon chopped dill, plus extra to serve

1 tablespoon chopped chives, plus extra to serve

½ teaspoon ground allspice

pinch of ground nutmeg

400g (14oz) can chopped tomatoes

1 tablespoon caraway seeds

1 tablespoon paprika

1 tablespoon red pepper paste

250ml (9fl oz) chicken stock

salt and pepper

150g (5½oz) thick Greek yogurt, to serve

1 Going in from the base of the cabbage, remove the core. Blanch the cabbage in boiling salted water for 2–3 minutes. Drain and refresh in running cold water. Remove 12 of the larger leaves and set aside. Roughly chop the smaller leaves.

2 Spread half of the sauerkraut over the base of an ovenproof dish with the chopped cabbage. Mix the minced turkey with the ricotta and beaten egg. In a small pan, heat half the olive oil with half the onions and garlic for 5 minutes to soften. When cool, add to the turkey mix along with the herbs, allspice and nutmeg. Season and mix well.

3 Lay out the 12 cabbage leaves on a chopping board or clean work surface. Divide the turkey mix between each leaf and roll each leaf into a small parcel. Place each parcel on top of the chopped cabbage in the baking dish.

4 Preheat the oven to 180°C (350°F/gas mark 4).

5 In the same pan, cook the remaining onion and garlic in the remaining oil for 5 minutes. Add the tomatoes with the spices and red pepper paste. Mix well and simmer for 10 minutes, then add the stock and the remaining sauerkraut. Season and pour over the cabbage parcels.

6 Bake for 40 minutes. Serve with the yogurt and extra chopped dill and chives.

Chicken with coriander, lemon & spinach

Cooked chard or spring greens can be used instead of spinach. Another dish which can be served with Raita (page 176) and Kachumber (page 118).

Serves 4

3 tablespoons olive oil

8 skinless, boneless chicken thighs

1 onion, finely chopped

2 teaspoons grated fresh ginger

4 garlic cloves, crushed

1 green chilli, deseeded and chopped

2 teaspoons ground cumin

1 teaspoon ground coriander

½ teaspoon ground turmeric

100g (3½oz) coriander, chopped

juice of 1 lemon

150ml (5fl oz) chicken stock

250g (9oz) spinach

salt and pepper

1 Heat 2 tablespoons of oil in a large, shallow pan. Brown the chicken thighs on both sides and season with salt and pepper. Remove from the pan with a slotted spoon and set aside.

2 Add the onion to the pan and cook gently for 10 minutes to soften. Add the ginger, garlic and chilli. Cook for 2 minutes, then add all the spices and fresh coriander. Stir well, then add the lemon juice and stock. Return the chicken to the pan and bring to a simmer, then reduce the heat and cook slowly for about 20 minutes or until the chicken is tender.

3 While the chicken is cooking, heat the remaining tablespoon of oil in a large pan. Add the spinach to the hot oil and stir quickly to wilt. Season well, drain in a colander and roughly chop.

4 Add the spinach to the cooked chicken and stir to combine. Serve with Raita (page 176) and Kachumber (page 118).

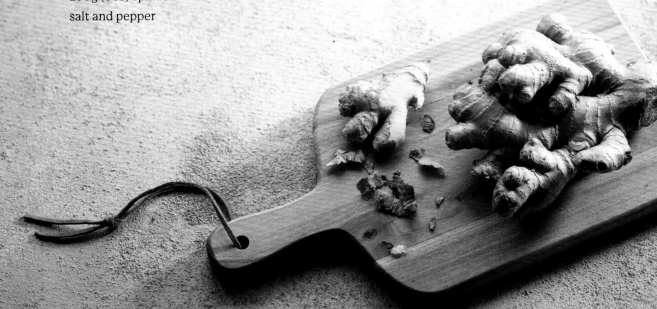

Venison ragout

Perfect ragout for pasta. Choose fresh egg pappardelle or a good buckwheat tagliatelle and have a peppery rocket salad to start.

Serves 6

10g (¼oz) dried porcini, soaked in 100ml (3½fl oz) boiling water

3 tablespoons olive oil

500g (1lb 2oz) minced venison

1 onion, chopped

2 celery sticks, chopped

1 large carrot, peeled and chopped

1 leek, chopped

3 garlic cloves, crushed

1 tablespoon chopped rosemary

1 sprig of thyme

200ml (7fl oz) red wine

400g (14oz) can chopped tomatoes

1 tablespoon tomato purée (or red pepper paste)

300ml (10fl oz) chicken stock

2 tablespoons chopped flat leaf parsley

salt and pepper

1 Drain the porcini, reserving the soaking liquor, and chop the mushrooms.

2 Heat the oil in large pan and brown the venison mince in batches. Season, then remove with a slotted spoon and set aside. Add the onion, celery, carrot and leek and cook over a gentle heat for 10 minutes.

3 Add the chopped porcini, garlic and herbs and cook for a minute, then pour in the red wine. Stir well and cook over a high heat for 2 minutes. Return the venison to the pan with the chopped tomatoes, porcini soaking liquor, tomato purée and stock. Stir well and simmer for about 1 hour, topping up with more stock or water if the sauce becomes dry.

4 Season well and stir through the chopped parsley.

Venison is particularly rich in iron and contains more protein than any other red meat.

Spiced chicken with red pepper & almond sauce

A very easy curry based on an early Madhur Jaffrey recipe. Serve with Raita (page 176) and Kachumber (page 118).

Serves 4

2 tablespoons coconut or olive oil

8 skinless, boneless chicken thighs

250ml (9fl oz) chicken stock

juice of ½ lemon

salt and pepper

chopped coriander, to serve

Paste

1 red onion, roughly chopped

2 red peppers, deseeded and chopped

1 tablespoon chopped fresh ginger

4 garlic cloves, crushed

2 teaspoons red pepper paste

2 teaspoons ground cumin

1 teaspoon ground coriander

1 teaspoon ground turmeric

75g (2½oz) flaked almonds (or ground almonds)

1 red chilli

1 In a food processor, blitz all the paste ingredients to make a smooth paste, adding a little water to help the ingredients break down.

2 Heat the oil in a large, shallow pan and add the red pepper paste. Stir well and fry over a low heat for about 15 minutes. While the paste is cooking, cut each chicken thigh into 3 pieces. Add the chicken to the paste and cook for another 5 minutes over a high heat, coating the chicken and stirring constantly to stop the paste catching.

3 Add the chicken stock and bring to the boil. Simmer gently over a low heat for 15 minutes or until the chicken is cooked.

4 Add the lemon juice and season well. Serve sprinkled with chopped coriander.

All colours of pepper are a rich source of vitamins C and A, but red peppers contain the highest amounts of polyphenols and carotenes.

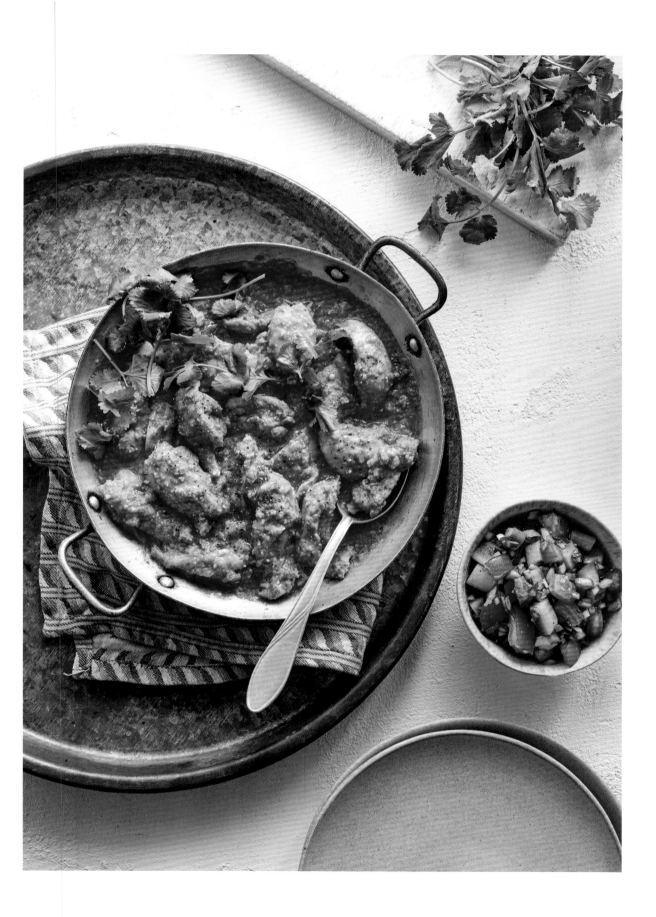

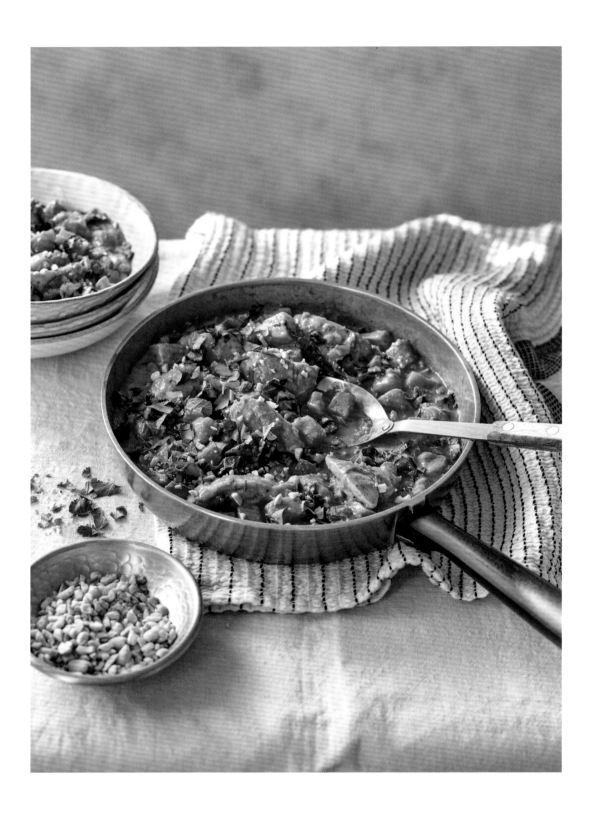

Sweet potato stew with chicken, peanuts & spring greens

A hearty, lightly spiced stew. Use chard or kale instead of spring greens if you prefer. The combination of ingredients in this recipe makes it nature's multi-vitamin!

Serves 4

2 tablespoons olive oil

4 skinless, boneless chicken thighs, each cut into 3 pieces

1 onion, finely chopped

2 teaspoons grated fresh ginger

3 garlic cloves, crushed

1 red pepper, deseeded and chopped

2 sweet potatoes, peeled and cut into rough 1cm (½in) pieces

1 teaspoon ground cumin

½ teaspoon ground turmeric

pinch of ground cinnamon

1 teaspoon smoked paprika

½ teaspoon dried oregano

200g (7oz) canned chopped tomatoes

300ml (10fl oz) chicken stock

100g (3½oz) spring greens, deveined and shredded

75g (2½oz) smooth peanut butter

1 tablespoon apple cider vinegar

2 tablespoons crushed toasted peanuts

2 tablespoons chopped coriander

salt and pepper

1 Heat the oil in a large, shallow pan. Season the chicken pieces and fry in batches until browned on both sides. Remove with a slotted spoon and set aside.

2 Add the chopped onion to the same pan and cook for 10 minutes to soften before adding the ginger, garlic and red pepper. Cook for 2 minutes before adding the diced sweet potato and all the spices and oregano. Season and stir well.

3 Stir in the chopped tomatoes and cook for 5 minutes, then add the stock. Turn up the heat and bring to a simmer, adding the chicken. Reduce the heat and cook gently for about 15 minutes until the sweet potato is soft and the chicken is cooked through.

4 Place the shredded spring greens on top of the stew, cover the pan and allow to steam for 5 minutes. Stir through the peanut butter and the vinegar, adding more water or stock if needed. Season well.

5 Serve sprinkle with toasted peanuts and chopped coriander.

Chicken and summer veg with a grape & tarragon dressing

A lovely fresh dish using seasonal greens and loads of tarragon.

Serves 4

4 skin on, boneless chicken thighs

1 leek, thinly sliced

1 tablespoon olive oil

100g (3½oz) French beans

100g (3½oz) runner beans, sliced

100g (3½oz) frozen peas

100g (3½oz) sugar snap peas, thinly sliced

100g (3½oz) cooked artichokes, thinly sliced

100g (3½oz) flageolet beans (or other white beans, canned or cooked from dried beans)

1 small bunch of chard, leaves thinly sliced

salt and pepper

Dressing

2 tablespoons chopped tarragon

1 banana shallot, finely chopped

2 tablespoons moscatel vinegar

2 teaspoons maple syrup

10 green or red grapes, thinly sliced

4 tablespoons rapeseed oil

1 Macerate the tarragon with the shallots in the vinegar, maple syrup and the grapes for about 1 hour. Stir in the oil.

2 Season the chicken thighs well. Heat a large, shallow, non-stick frying pan and add the chicken thighs, skin-side down. Cook for about 10 minutes over a low heat to render out the fat. Flip the thighs over and cook for another 10 minutes. Set aside to rest.

3 Cook the leek in the oil for 5 minutes until tender. Bring a large pan of salted water to the boil. Tip in the French and runner beans and cook for 2 minutes over a high heat. Add the peas and bring back to the boil. Check the beans are tender, then drain.

4 Tip the drained beans into a bowl with the leek, sugar snap peas, sliced artichokes, white beans and chard. Toss together with the tarragon dressing and top with sliced chicken thighs.

Chicken is a great source of protein and choline as well as iron and vitamin B12.

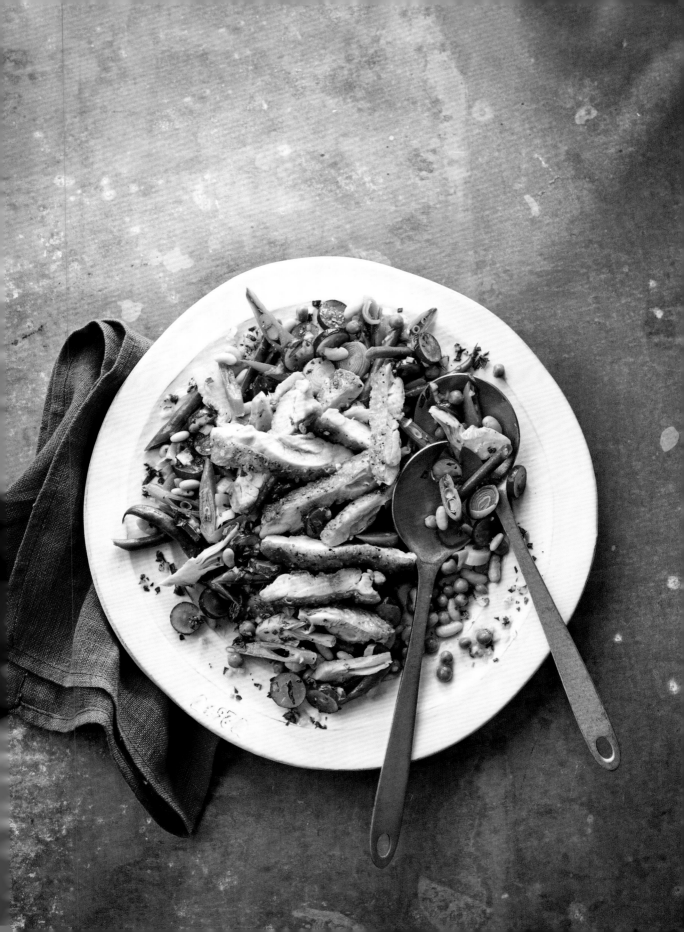

Sides, Sauces & Snacks

7

Raita

An essential side for an Indian curry, of which there are many variations. Grated carrot can be added instead of beetroot. This also makes a delicious and refreshing dip that is perfect with salad or chopped raw vegetables. The natural Greek yogurt is a great probiotic food and the fresh mint and cumin seeds are both high in helpful polyphenols.

Serves 4

250g (9oz) Greek yogurt

2 shallots, finely chopped

½ cucumber, peeled, deseeded and grated

½ teaspoon toasted ground cumin seeds

1–2 tablespoons chopped mint

salt and pepper

1   Mix all the ingredients together and season.

Beetroot raita

To 250g (9oz) yogurt, add salt, ground cumin and chopped green chilli. Grate a small raw beetroot and stir into the raita. In a small frying pan, heat 1 tablespoon of olive oil. Add 1 teaspoon of black mustard seeds, 10 curry leaves and 1 teaspoon of split urad dal. When the mustard seeds start to pop, turn off the heat and pour onto the purple raita.

Pickled cucumber

This keeps in the fridge for a few weeks and is a great addition to lots of dishes. Add more chilli for a spicier result.

Serves 4-6

2 cucumbers

1 teaspoon salt

1 tablespoon caster sugar

3 tablespoons rice vinegar

2 tablespoons sesame seeds

1 teaspoon chilli flakes

3 tablespoons sunflower oil

1   Peel the skin of the cucumber running down the length of it to leave a few stripes of green skin. Cut the cucumber in half lengthways and scoop out the seeds. Finely slice each half to make half-moons. Toss with the salt and leave in a colander for at least 30 minutes to drain excess water.

2   Dry with kitchen paper and place in a dry bowl. Mix with the sugar and vinegar and taste to achieve your desired sweet and sour flavour. Add more sugar or vinegar if required.

3   Toast the sesame seeds and chilli flakes in the oil until the seeds start to colour. Immediately tip into the cucumber and stir well. This can be made up to 2 days in advance as the flavours will improve over time.

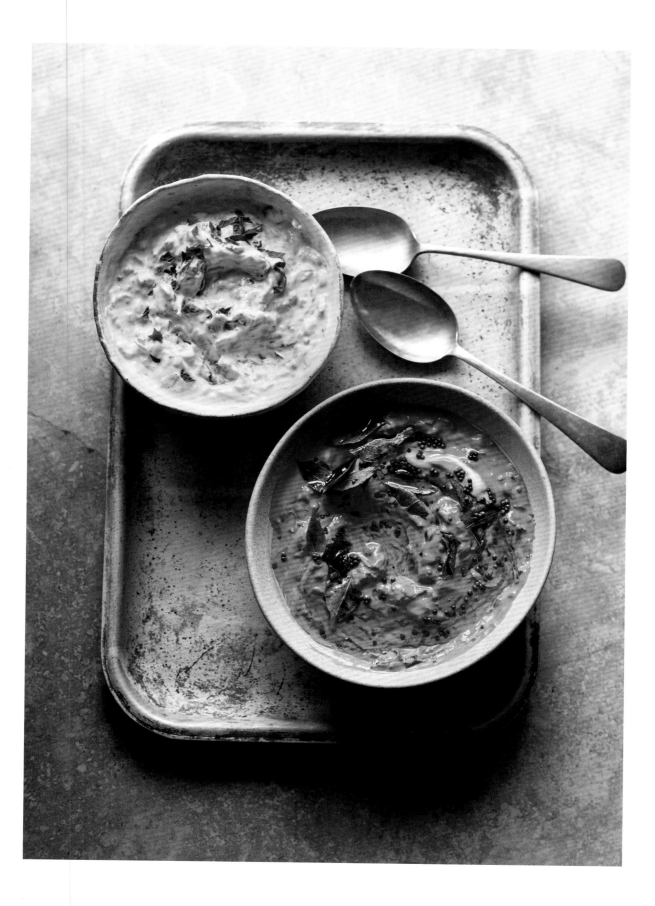

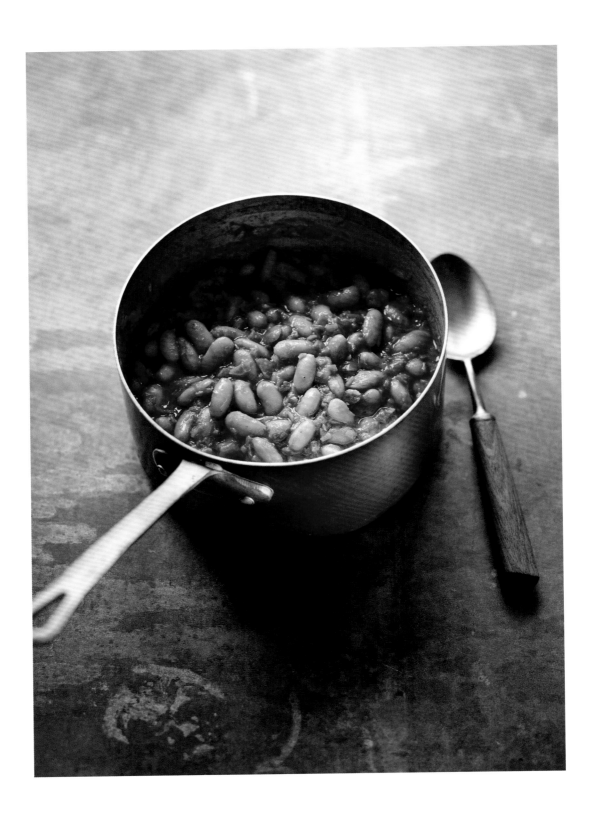

My Boston baked beans

Home-cooked white beans have a far better flavour than canned white beans. If you are using canned beans, rinse them really well. This makes a brilliant side or you can serve it on nutty bread for a delicious fibre- and protein-packed plant-based breakfast.

Serves 4–6

3 tablespoons olive oil

1 onion, finely chopped

2 celery sticks, finely chopped

1 leek, finely chopped

3 garlic cloves, crushed

200g (7oz) canned chopped tomatoes (or passata)

1 heaped tablespoon red pepper paste

1 teaspoon smoked paprika

400g (14oz) haricot or cannellini beans (canned or cooked from dried beans)

1 tablespoon Dijon or English mustard

Worcestershire sauce, to taste

Tabasco sauce, to taste

2 teaspoons molasses sugar

2 teaspoons balsamic vinegar

salt and pepper

1   Heat the oil in a large pan and add the chopped vegetables. Cook over a medium heat for 15 minutes without colouring the veg. Add the garlic and cook for 2 minutes before tipping in the tomatoes, followed by the red pepper paste and paprika. Simmer gently for another 15 minutes until the sauce has reduced without catching.

2   Add the cooked beans and stir well. Bring to a simmer and add the remaining ingredients. Stir in 150ml (5fl oz) of water. Simmer for another 10 minutes and season well.

Serve on grilled rye sourdough or with poached eggs.

Tomatoes contain lycopene; the red-tinged plant chemical that has a protective effect on the body helping to repair and reduce oxidation. Cooking tomatoes makes the lycopene more absorbable.

Dr Fede's spice mix

This delivers a delicious combination of flavour and beneficial spices for better wellbeing. Add to scrambled eggs, grilled meat or fish and to season grains.

Makes a small (200g) jar

1 teaspoon ground turmeric

1 teaspoon ground black pepper

2 teaspoons dried oregano

2 teaspoons dried marjoram

1 teaspoon ground cumin

3 teaspoons ground flax seeds

2 teaspoons chaga mushroom powder (optional)

1 Mix all the ingredients together and store in an airtight container/jar for 4 weeks.

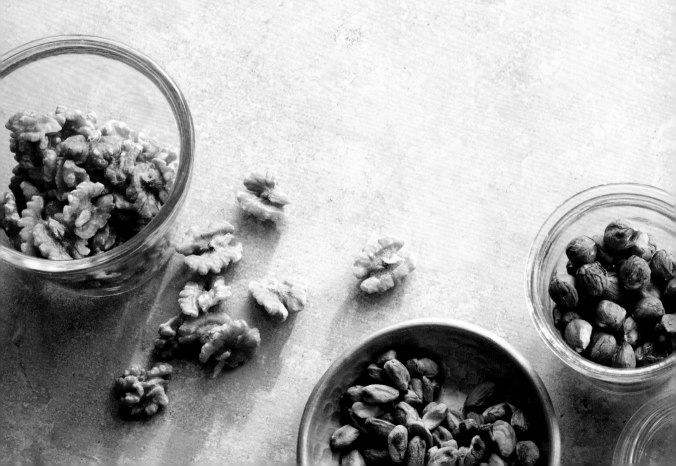

Trail mix

A favourite of Dr Fede's, this is the perfect snack to keep in a Kilner jar on the kitchen side. The combination of nuts, seeds and apricot is great for heart health and makes for a tasty addition to meals or snack on the go. Any nuts can be used. Toasting them first improves the flavour and texture.

Makes 450g (1lb) jar

100g (3½oz) walnut pieces

100g (3½oz) flaked almonds

75g (2½oz) pumpkin seeds

75g (2½oz) pistachios

100g (3½oz) dried apricots, sliced

1　Preheat the oven to 160°C (325°F/gas mark 3).

2　Place the walnuts, almonds and pumpkin seeds on a baking tray and roast lightly for 5-10 minutes. Leave to cool.

3　Mix the cooled walnuts, almonds and pumpkin seeds with the pistachios and apricots. Keep in a sealed container for up to 4 weeks.

Seed mix

This can be sprinkled on eggs, salads and soups for texture and flavour.

Makes 500g (1lb 2oz)

150g (5½oz) pumpkin seeds

150g (5½oz) sunflower seeds

100g (3½oz) flax seeds

75g (2½oz) sesame seeds

75g (2½oz) hemp seeds

1　Preheat the oven to 160°C (325°F/gas mark 3).

2　Roast the seeds in the oven separately. The larger seeds will take longer than the smaller ones. Check after 10 minutes and remove the toasted seeds, When all are lightly roasted, leave to cool.

3　Mix all the seeds together and store in an airtight container for up to 4 weeks .

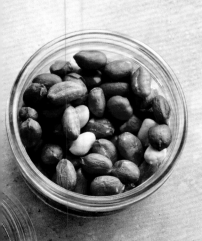

Seedy nutty bread

This bread toasts really well and is a good gluten-free option. It is full of fibre, plant protein and polyphenols, making it great for your gut health as well as providing a variety of nutrients found in the seeds and nuts.

Makes 1 loaf

70g (2½oz) pumpkin seeds

70g (2½oz) sunflower seeds

50g (1¾oz) sesame seeds

100g (3½oz) ground almonds

100g (3½oz) buckwheat flour

100g (3½oz) gluten-free oats

50g (1¾oz) flax seeds

2 tablespoons psyllium husks

2 tablespoons ground chia seeds

1½ teaspoons salt

50ml (2fl oz) olive oil

2 tablespoons maple syrup

500ml (18fl oz) water

1 Preheat the oven to 170°C (340°F/gas mark 3½). Line a 900g (2lb) loaf tin wiith baking parchment.

2 Roast the pumpkin seeds, sunflower seeds and sesame seeds on a baking tray for 10–15 minutes or until the seeds are lightly coloured. Leave to cool and mix in a large bowl with the remaining dry ingredients.

3 Whisk the remaining (wet) ingredients together and pour into the dry. Beat well to combine. Pour into the lined loaf tin. Cover and leave overnight in the fridge.

4 Preheat the oven to 200°C (400°F/gas mark 6).

5 Remove the loaf from the fridge and allow it to come up to room temperature. Bake for 50 minutes–1 hour. Leave to cool on a wire rack before slicing. This loaf keeps for a few days in an airtight container.

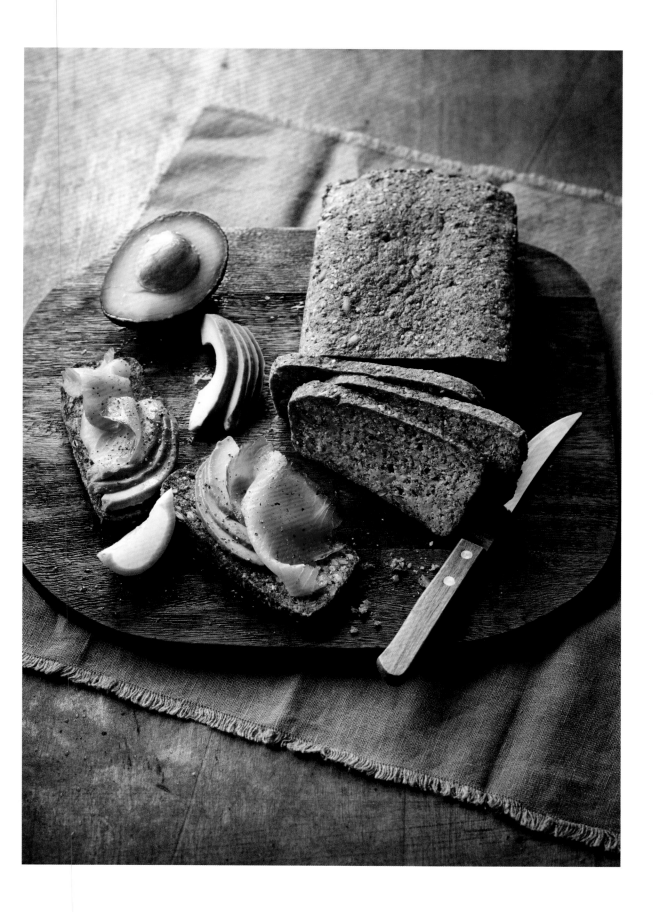

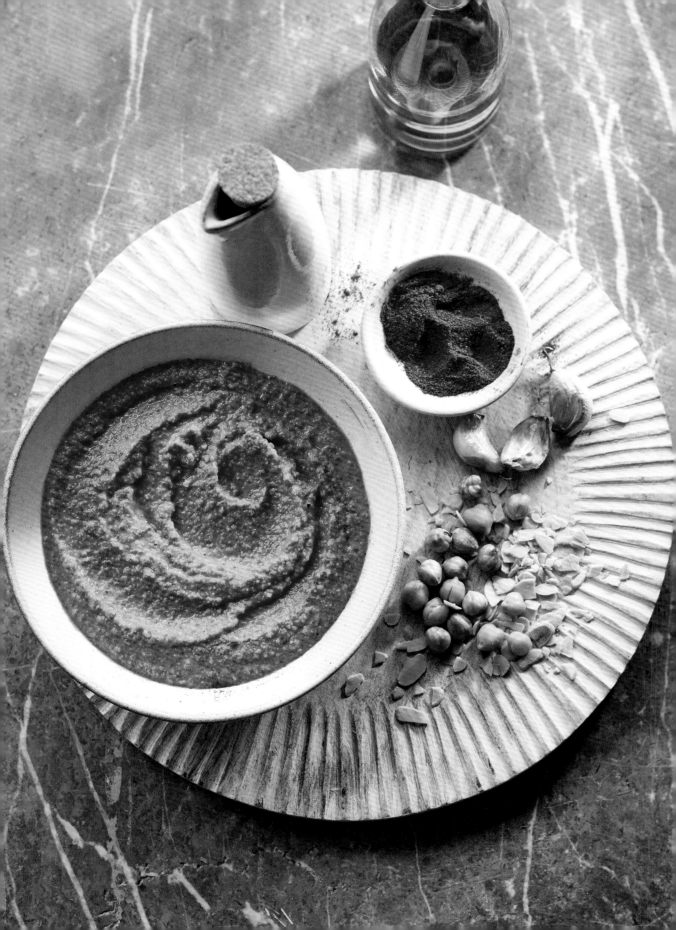

Romesco sauce

The addition of chickpeas instead of bread makes a creamier sauce with added fibre and plant protein to boot. Lovely with roasted vegetables and grilled fish.

Serves 4–6

4 tomatoes

12 garlic cloves, unpeeled

50g (1¾oz) flaked almonds

50g (1¾oz) blanched hazelnuts

200g (7oz) piquillo or peeled roasted red peppers

3 tablespoons cooked chickpeas

2 teaspoons paprika

50ml (2fl oz) sherry vinegar

pinch of cayenne pepper

150ml (5fl oz) olive oil

salt and pepper

1 Preheat the oven to 180°C (350°F/gas mark 4).

2 Roast the tomatoes with the garlic for about 20 minutes until the tomatoes are slightly charred and the garlic is soft. Roast the nuts in the oven for 5 minutes until lightly browned.

3 Squeeze the flesh from the garlic and place in a food processor with the roasted tomatoes. Add the remaining ingredients, except the olive oil, and blitz to a paste. Pour in the olive oil with the motor running until you have a smooth paste, adding a little water if necessary. Season to taste. The sauce keeps well in a sealed container in the fridge for up to 5 days.

Kimchi miso mayonnaise

A great vegan mayonnaise that is popular with everyone. Quick to make and a good dipping sauce or with grilled fish and seafood. As the miso is a fermented food, it adds good bacteria to boost your gut health.

Serves 6

2 heaped tablespoons kimchi

3 tablespoons white miso paste

100g (3½oz) silken tofu

1 tablespoon sesame oil

2 tablespoons rice vinegar

2 teaspoons maple syrup

100ml (3½fl oz) flavourless oil

1 Place all the ingredients except the oil in a food processor and blitz to make a coarse purée. Slowly add the oil to emulsify, making a thick mayonnaise. The mayonnaise keeps well in a sealed container in the fridge for up to 7 days.

Kale and nut pesto

A good pasta sauce. Add a little of the pasta cooking water to the pesto to get a better coating consistency.

Serves 4

100g (3½oz) kale leaves, chopped

1 small bunch of basil, leaves picked

zest and juice of 1 lemon

2 tablespoons walnuts, toasted

2 tablespoons pine nuts, toasted

3 garlic cloves, crushed

50g (1¾oz) grated Parmesan or pecorino

75ml (2½fl oz) olive oil

1 tomato, roughly chopped

salt and pepper

1 Place all the ingredients in a liquidizer or powerful food processor. Blitz until it becomes a thick paste, adding a little water if needed.

Extra virgin olive oil is full of healthy poly-unsaturated fats and plant antioxidants, it is shown to protect against inflammation, heart disease, breast cancer and type 2 diabetes. The only real super food to add on every occasion!

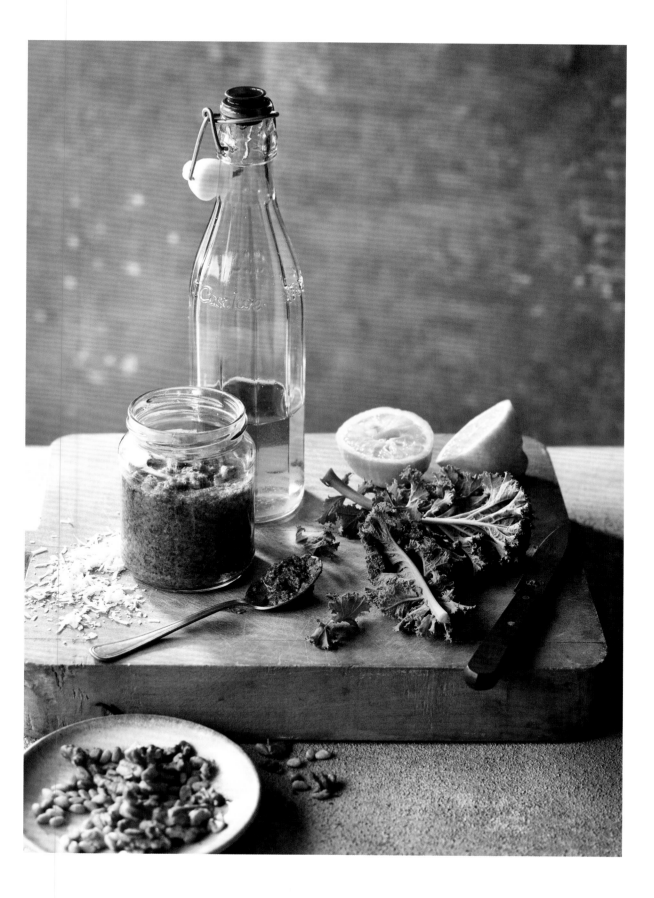

Desserts

8

Grilled peaches with raspberries, yogurt & almonds

A lighter and healthier version of a peach Melba, though with a little booze added. When peaches are in season, this simple dessert is heavenly. The Greek yogurt and raspberries add protein, fats and fibre to create balance to this sweet dessert.

Serves 4

4 ripe peaches, halved and stoned

1 tablespoon olive oil

1 tablespoon maple syrup (optional)

300g (10½oz) raspberries

3 tablespoons icing sugar (optional)

juice of 1 orange

100g (3½oz) flaked almonds

200g (7oz) Greek yogurt

1 teaspoon vanilla extract

50ml (2fl oz) Amaretto, brandy or grappa (optional)

1 Preheat the oven to 170°C (340°F/gas mark 3½).

2 Heat a griddle pan (or non-stick frying pan) over a medium heat. Rub the cut side of the peaches with the olive oil and place the peaches in the pan, cut-side down. Cook for a few minutes over a medium heat until the cut side is lightly browned.

3 Flip the peaches over and brush the cut side with the maple syrup if you like. Cook for another 3—4 minutes over a low heat or until the peaches are cooked but not mushy. Set aside.

4 Place 200g (7oz) of the raspberries in a blender with half the icing sugar (if using) and the orange juice. Blend until smooth, adding a little water so you have the consistency of double cream. Strain for a smooth sauce.

5 Toss the flaked almonds with the remaining icing sugar (if using). Spread out on a lined baking tray and bake in the oven for about 10 minutes or until the almonds are lightly browned.

6 Mix the yogurt with the vanilla extract. To serve, top the peach halves with yogurt, drizzle with the raspberry sauce and Amaretto. Sprinkle with the remaining raspberries and toasted almonds. The peaches can be served warm or at room temperature.

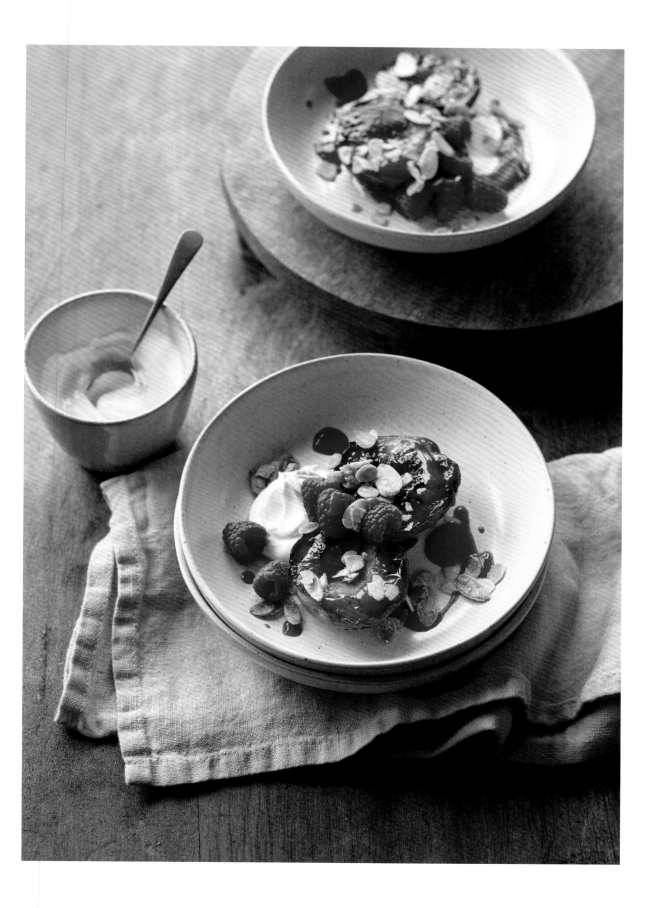

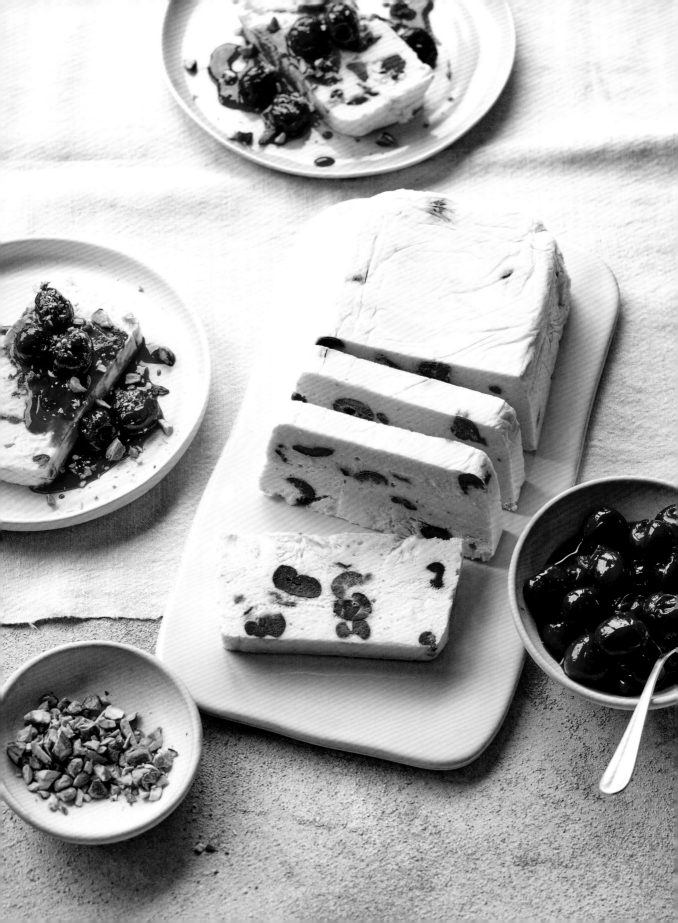

Yogurt semifreddo with cherries & pistachios

Yogurt and cherries make for a delicious combination and you can add kefir for an added probiotic hit. Any other cooked fruit can be added to the yogurt base. Rhubarb would work particularly well, as would any soft fruit.

Serves 6–8

4 egg whites

150g (5½oz) honey

pinch of cream of tartar

pinch of salt

500g (1lb 2oz) Greek yogurt

pinch of ground cardamom

zest of 1 orange

½ teaspoon vanilla extract

150g (5½oz) frozen cherries (or cherry halves)

300g (10½oz) cherries, pitted

50g (1¾oz) caster sugar

50ml (2fl oz) cherry brandy

75g (2½oz) pistachios, chopped

1 Line a 900g (2lb) loaf tin with baking parchment.

2 In a large bowl over a pan of simmering water, whisk the egg whites lightly with the honey, cream of tartar and salt. Simmer for about 3 minutes until the honey has dissolved and the mixture is warm. Take off the heat and whisk well for 5 minutes until the meringue is glossy and stiff.

3 In a large bowl, mix the yogurt with the cardamom, orange zest and vanilla extract. Whisk in a quarter of the meringue mixture and then carefully fold through the rest. Fold in the frozen cherries and spoon into the lined loaf tin. Cover and freeze for a minimum of 6 hours or overnight.

4 In a small pan, heat the fresh cherries with the sugar, cherry brandy and 50ml (2fl oz) water. Cook for about 5 minutes until the liquid has reduced and you have a thick sauce.

5 To serve, place slices of the semifreddo on a serving dish. Spoon over the sauce and sprinkle with pistachios.

Banana 'nice' cream

A brilliant way to reduce food waste and make an instant delicious and creamy dessert. Serve with added cacao powder, chopped nuts or berries.

Serves 4

4 very ripe bananas

A nut butter of your choice

Variations

Add cacao powder for a
chocolate flavour

Optional toppings

One chopped date

1 teaspoon coconut flakes

1 handful chopped walnuts

1 Peel the bananas and slice across. Put the sliced bananas in one layer on a lined tray in the freezer overnight.

2 Blitz the frozen bananas in a food processor until smooth, adding a nut butter of your choice. Instant ice cream!

Bananas are high in fibre and contain rich amounts of potassium, which can help reduce blood pressure and improve sleep quality.

Plum, blueberry & oat crumble

Plums and blueberries are rich in brilliant polyphenols and this simple twist on a classic dessert is a warming and nutritious end to a meal. The hazelnuts and almonds add fibre and protein as well as crunch and depth of flavour.

Serves 6

1kg (2lb 4oz) plums, stoned and cut into 2cm (¾in) pieces

200g (7oz) blueberries

2 tablespoons light soft brown sugar

zest and juice of 1 orange

3 tablespoons rum

Crumble

75g (2½oz) ground hazelnuts

50g flaked almonds, roughly chopped

50g (1¾oz) plain flour

75g (2½oz) steel-cut oats

50g (1¾oz) light soft brown sugar

100g (3½oz) unsalted butter

1 Preheat the oven to 160°C (325°F/gas mark 3).

2 Mix the plums with the blueberries, sugar, orange zest and juice and rum. Place in a ovenproof dish so the fruit is roughly 2cm (¾in) deep.

3 In a large bowl, mix the dry ingredients together and cut the butter into small squares. Using your fingertips, rub the butter into the mixture so it resembles chunky breadcrumbs. Alternatively, this can be done in a food processor.

4 Sprinkle the crumble mixture over the fruit and bake for 30–40 minutes until the top is brown and the fruit juices are bubbling around the sides of the dish.

5 Serve with Greek yogurt if you like.

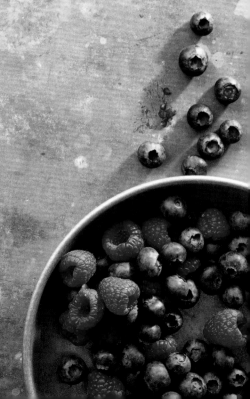

Fruit salad with mint & almonds

The best way to enjoy fruit is at the end of a meal, and fruit salads are a delicious way to make it interesting and colourful. Serve with mint and almonds for added flavour and texture.

Serves 4

zest and juice of 1 lemon

3 tablespoons limoncello (optional)

1 tablespoon honey (optional)

2 tablespoons shredded mint leaves

½ melon, flesh cubed

1 peach, stoned and sliced

150g (5½oz) raspberries

150g (5½oz) strawberries, quartered

2 apples, cored and diced

75g (2½oz) flaked almonds, toasted

1   Mix the lemon zest and juice, limoncello and honey with the mint. Whisk well in a large bowl. Tip in the prepared fruit and toss through the dressing

2   Serve sprinkled with toasted almonds.

Strawberries are packed with antioxidants and rich in vitamin C.

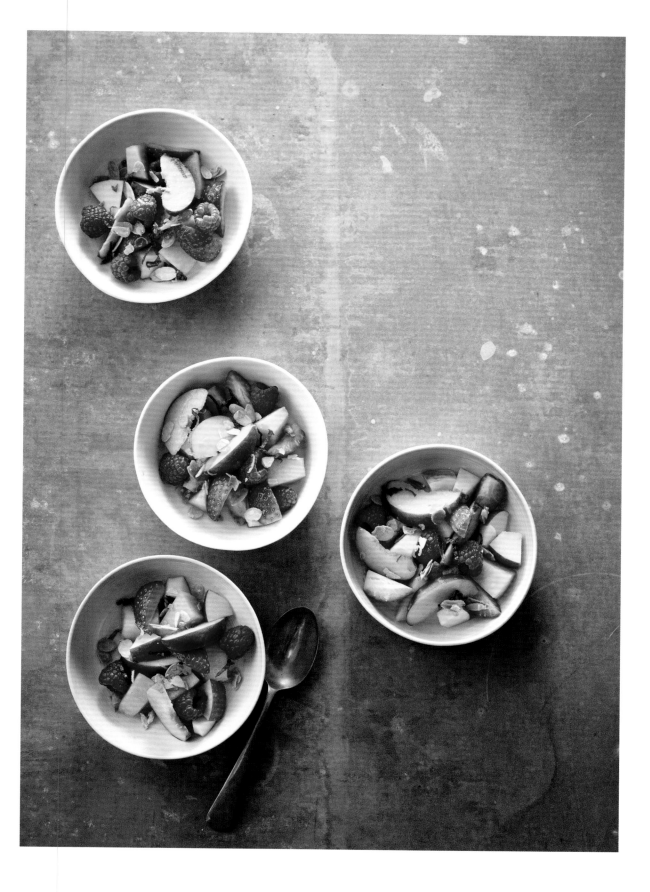

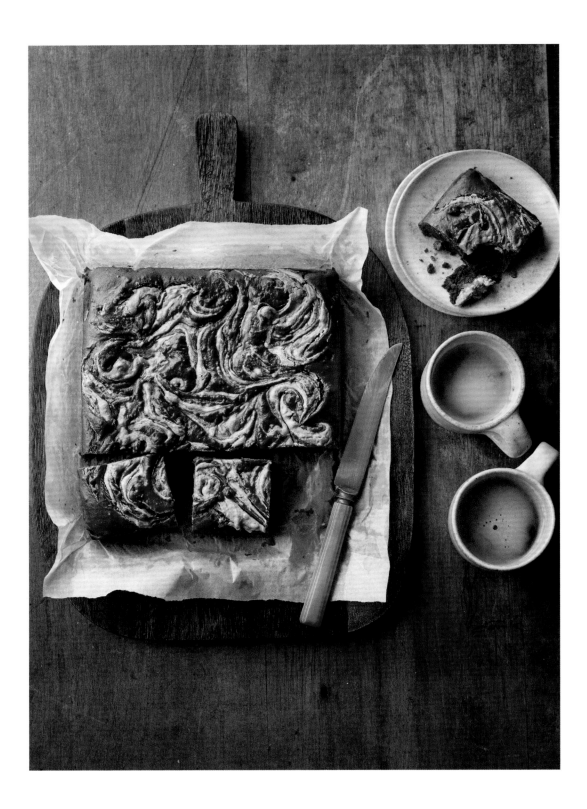

Chocolate, peanut butter & banana brownies

Very quick and easy to make in a food processor. Adding peanut butter, ground almonds and pecans with dark chocolate makes a delicious and nutritious dessert. Enjoy at the end of a meal with some fresh berries.

Makes 9–12

2 large, ripe bananas, peeled

250g (9oz) smooth peanut butter, plus extra to decorate

80g (2¾oz) maple syrup

2 eggs

20g (¾oz) cocoa powder

20g (¾oz) ground almonds

1 teaspoon vanilla extract

1 teaspoon bicarbonate of soda

½ teaspoon baking powder

100g (3½oz) dark chocolate chips

100g (3½oz) pecans, roughly chopped

1 Preheat the oven to 160°C (325°F/gas mark 3). Line a 20cm (8in) square cake tin with baking parchment.

2 In a food processor, blend the bananas with the peanut butter, maple syrup and eggs until smooth. Mix together the remaining ingredients. Fold the dry ingredients into the wet. Spoon the mixture into the lined baking tin.

3 Swirl the extra peanut butter on top of the cake mix and bake for 20–25 minutes or until a skewer inserted into the centre comes out clean. Leave in the tin for 5 minutes, then leave to cool on a wire rack, before cutting into 9 or 12 brownies. These should keep in an airtight container for up to 3-4 days.

Dark (70% cocoa solids) chocolate is a good source of iron, magnesium, copper, manganese, potassium, phosphorus, zinc and selenium.

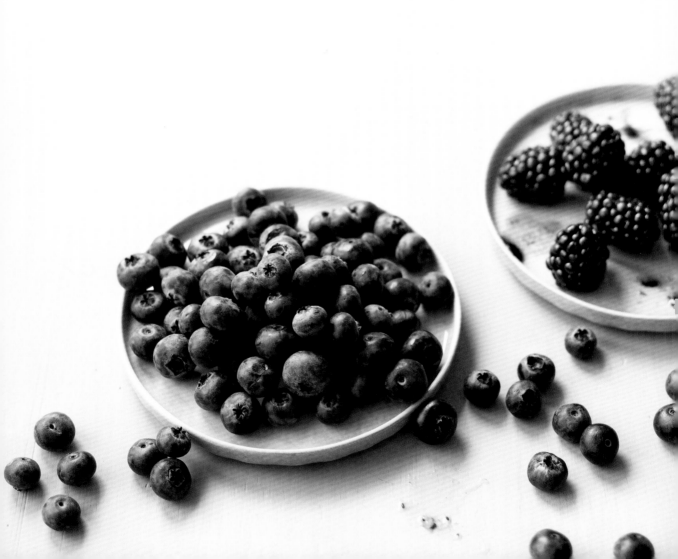

Endnotes

1 International Agency for Research on Cancer, EPIC Study. https://epic.iarc.fr/about/about.php

2 World Health Organization. https://www.who.int/news-room/fact-sheets/detail/noncommunicable-diseases

3 World Health Organization, Global Status Report. https://apps.who.int/iris/handle/10665/148114

4 Rawaf S., Amati F., McDonald A., Majeed A., Dubois E., Implementation and Evaluation of Patient-centred Care in Experimental Studies from 2000-2010: Systematic Review, *International Journal of Person Centred Medicine*, 2017. http://ijpcm.org/index.php/ijpcm/article/view/77

5 Lee K., Ferry A., Anand A., et al., Sex-Specific Thresholds of High-Sensitivity Troponin in Patients With Suspected Acute Coronary Syndrome, *Journal of the American College of Cardiology*, 2019. https://www.jacc.org/doi/10.1016/j.jacc.2019.07.082

6 Amati F., Hassounah S., Swaka A., The Impact of Mediterranean Dietary Patterns During Pregnancy on Maternal and Offspring Health, *Nutrients*, 2019. https://www.mdpi.com/2072-6643/11/5/1098

7 Women's Health Concern, HRT: Benefits and Risks. https://www.womens-health-concern.org/wp-content/uploads/2022/12/11-WHC-FACTSHEET-HRT-BenefitsRisks-NOV2022-B.pdf

8 Women's Health Concern, Understanding the Risks of Breast Cancer. https://www.womens-health-concern.org/wp-content/uploads/2019/10/WHC-UnderstandingRisksofBreastCancer-MARCH2017.pdf

9 Zheng P., Zeng B., Zhou C. et al., Gut Microbiome Remodeling Induces Depressive-like Behaviors Through a Pathway Mediated by the Host's Metabolism, *Molecular Psychiatry*, 2016. https://www.nature.com/articles/mp201644

10 Fabbri A., Holland T.J., Bero L.A., Food Industry Sponsorship of Academic Research: Investigating Commercial Bias in the Research Agenda, *Public Health Nutrition*, 2018. https://pubmed.ncbi.nlm.nih.gov/30157979/

11 Snieder H., MacGregor A.J., Spector T.D., Genes Control the Cessation of a Woman's Reproductive Life: A Twin Study of Hysterectomy and Age at Menopause, *The Journal of Clinical Endocrinology & Metabolism*, 1998. https://academic.oup.com/jcem/article/83/6/1875/2865177

12 Shanley D.P., Sear R., Mace R., Kirkwood T.B.L, Testing Evolutionary Theories of Menopause, *National Library of Medicine*, 2007. ncbi.nlm.nih.gov/pmc/articles/PMC2291159/

13 Anagnostis P., Christou K., Artzouchaltzi A., Gkekas N.K., Kosmidou N., Siolos P., Paschou S.A., et al., Early Menopause and Premature Ovarian Insufficiency are Associated with Increased Risk of Type 2 Diabetes: A Systematic Review and Meta-analysis, *European Journal of Endocrinology*, 2019. https://rb.gy/wv8k5

14 E Zhu D., Chung H-F., Dobson A.J., Pandeya N., Giles G.G., Bruinsma F., et al., Age at Natural Menopause and Risk of Incident Cardiovascular Disease: A Pooled Analysis of Individual Patient Data, *The Lancet*, 2019. https://doi.org/10.1016/S2468-2667(19)30155-0

15 Appiah D., PhD, MPH1, Nwabuo C.C., MD, MPH2, Ebong I.A. MD, MS3, et al., Trends in Age at Natural Menopause and Reproductive Life Span Among US Women, 1959-2018, *JAMA*, 2021. https://jamanetwork.com/journals/jama/fullarticle/2778126

16 Bulsara J., Patel P., Soni A., Acharya S., A Review: Brief Insight into Polycystic Ovarian Syndrome, *Endocrine and Metabolic Science*, 2021. https://www.sciencedirect.com/science/article/pii/S266639612100008X

17 Dunneram Y., Greenwood D.C., Burley V.J., Cade J.E., Dietary Intake and Age at Natural Menopause: Results from the UK Women's Cohort Study, *Journal of Epidemiology and Community Health*, 2018. 10.1136/jech-2017-209887

18 E Zhu D., Chung H-F., Pandeya N., et al., Body Mass Index and Age at Natural Menopause: An International Pooled Analysis of 11 Prospective Studies, *European Journal of Epidemiology*, 2017. https://link.springer.com/article/10.1007/s10654-018-0367-y

19 Britt K.L., Cuzick J. & Phillips K.A., Key Steps for Effective Breast Cancer Prevention, *Nat Rev Cancer*, 2020. https://doi.org/10.1038/s41568-020-0266-x

20 Podfigurna A., Meczekalski B., Functional Hypothalamic Amenorrhea: A Stress-Based Disease, *Endocrines*, 2021. https://www.mdpi.com/2673-396X/2/3/20

21 Arnot M., Emmott E.H., Mace R., The Relationship Between Social Support, Stressful Events, and Menopause Symptoms, *PLOS ONE*, 2021. https://doi.org/10.1371/journal.pone.0245444

22 Dunbar R.I.M., Breaking Bread: The Functions of Social Eating, *Adaptive Human Behavior and Physiology*, 2017. https://doi.org/10.1007/s40750-017-0061-4

23 Naito R., Leong D.P., Bangdiwala S.I., et al., Impact of Social Isolation on Mortality and Morbidity in 20 High-income, Middle-income and Low-income Countries in Five Continents, *BMJ Global Health*, 2021. https://gh.bmj.com/content/6/3/e004124

24 Cox C.E., Role of Physical Activity for Weight Loss and Weight Maintenance, *Diabetes Spectrum*, 2017. 10.2337/ds17-0013

25 Hall K.D., Kahan S., Maintenance of Lost Weight and Long-Term Management of Obesity, *Med Clin North Am*, 2018. 10.1016/j.mcna.2017.08.012

26 Butterfield D.A., Halliwell B., Oxidative stress, Dysfunctional Glucose Metabolism and Alzheimer Disease, *Nat Rev Neurosci*, 2019. https://doi.org/10.1038/s41583-019-0132-6

27 Cox C.E., Role of Physical Activity for Weight Loss and Weight Maintenance, *Diabetes Spectrum*, 2017. 10.2337/ds17-0013

28 Javadivala Z., Allahverdipour H., Jafarabadi M.A., Emam A., An Interventional Strategy of Physical Activity Promotion for Reduction of Menopause Symptoms, *Health Promot Perspect*, 2020. 10.34172/hpp.2020.57

• Endnotes •

29 Jacka F.N., O'Neil A., Opie R. et al., A Randomised Controlled Trial of Dietary Improvement for Adults with Major Depression (The 'SMILES' trial). *BMC Med*, 2017. https://doi.org/10.1186/s12916-017-0791-y

30 Martinez-Lacoba R., Pardo-Garcia I., Amo-Saus E., Escribano-Sotos F., Mediterranean Diet and Health Outcomes: A Systematic Meta-review, *European Journal of Public Health*, 2018. https://doi.org/10.1093/eurpub/cky113

31 Cano A., Marshall S., Zolfaroli I., et al., The Mediterranean Diet and Menopausal Health: An EMAS Position Statement, *Maturitas*, 2020. https://doi.org/10.1016/j.maturitas.2020.07.001

32 Herber-Gast G-C.M., Mishra G.D., Fruit, Mediterranean-style, and High-fat and -sugar Diets are Associated with the Risk of Night Sweats and Hot Flushes in Midlife: Results from a Prospective Cohort Study, *The American Journal of Clinical Nutrition*, 2013. https://doi.org/10.3945/ajcn.112.049965

33 Bermingham K.M, Linenberg I., Hall W.L., Kadé K., Franks P.W., Davies R., et al., Menopause is Associated with Postprandial Metabolism, Metabolic Health and Lifestyle: The ZOE PREDICT Study, *The Lancet*, https://doi.org/10.1016/j.ebiom.2022.104303

34 Nutt D.J., King, L.A., Phillips, L.D., Drug Harms in the UK: A Multicriteria Decision Analysis, *The Lancet*, 2010. https://doi.org/10.1016/S0140-6736(10)61462-6

35 McCaul M.E., Roach D., Hasin D.S., Weisner C., Chang G., Sinha R., Alcohol and Women: A Brief Overview, *Alcohol Clin Exp Res*, 2019. https://www.ncbi.nlm.nih.gov/pmc/articles/PMC6502688/

36 Castaldo L., Narváez A., Izzo L., Graziani G., Gaspari A., Minno G.D., Ritieni A., Red Wine Consumption and Cardiovascular Health, *Molecules*, 2019. https://www.ncbi.nlm.nih.gov/pmc/articles/PMC6804046/; Poli, A., Is Drinking Wine in Moderation Good for Health or Not?, *European Heart Journal Supplements*, 2022. https://doi.org/10.1093/eurheartjsupp/suac084

37 Landstra C.P., de Koning E.J.P., COVID-19 and Diabetes: Understanding the Interrelationship and Risks for a Severe Course, Front. *Endocrinol.*, 2021. https://doi.org/10.3389/fendo.2021.649525

38 PREDICT: The World's Largest In-depth Nutritional Research Program in the World, ZOE. https://joinzoe.com/post/what-is-predict

39 Loh M., Zhang W., Ng H.K. et al., Identification of Genetic Effects Underlying Type 2 Diabetes in South Asian and European Populations, *Commun Biol*, 2022. https://doi.org/10.1038/s42003-022-03248-5

40 Rohleder R., Stress and Inflammation – The Need to Address the Gap in the Transition Between Acute and Chronic Stress Effects, *Psychoneuroendocrinology*, 2019. https://doi.org/10.1016/j.psyneuen.2019.02.021

41 Marsh M.L., Oliveira M.N., Vieira-Potter V.J, Adipocyte Metabolism and Health after the Menopause: The Role of Exercise. *Nutrients*, 2023. https://doi.org/10.3390/nu15020444

42 Creedon A.C., Dimidi E., Hung E.S., Rossi M., Probert C., Grassby T., Miguens-Blanco J., Marchesi J.R., et al., The Impact of Almonds and Almond Processing on Gastrointestinal Physiology, Luminal Microbiology, and Gastrointestinal Symptoms: A Randomized Controlled Trial and Mastication Study, *The American Journal of Clinical Nutrition*, 2022. https://doi.org/10.1093/ajcn/nqac265

43 Vallat R., Berry S.E., Tsereteli N., et al., How people wake up is associated with previous night's sleep together with physical activity and food intake. *Nat Commun*, 2022. https://doi.org/10.1038/s41467-022-34503-2

44 Bermingham K.M., Linenberg I., Hall W.L., Kadé K., Franks P.W., Davies R., et al., Menopause is Associated With Postprandial Metabolism, Metabolic Health and Lifestyle: The ZOE PREDICT Study, The Lancet, 2022. https://doi.org/10.1016/j.ebiom.2022.104303

45 Amati F., McCann L.J., Spector T.D., The Gut Microbiome, Health and Personalised Nutrition, *Trends in Urology and Men's Health*, 2022. https://doi.org/10.1002/tre.856

46 Kwa M., Plottel C.S., Blaser M.J., Adams S., The Intestinal Microbiome and Estrogen Receptor-Positive Female Breast Cancer, *J Natl Cancer Inst*, 2016. https://www.ncbi.nlm.nih.gov/pmc/articles/PMC5017946/

47 Peters B.A., Lin J., Qi Q., Usyk M., Isasi C.R., Mossavar-Rahmani Y., Derby C.A., Santoro N., Perreira K.M., Daviglus M.L., Kominiarek M.A., Cai J., Knight R., Burk R.D., Kaplan R.C., Menopause Is Associated with an Altered Gut Microbiome and Estrobolome, with Implications for Adverse Cardiometabolic Risk in the Hispanic Community, Health Study/Study of Latinos, *mSystems*, 2022. https://www.ncbi.nlm.nih.gov/pmc/articles/PMC9239235/

48 Chen, L-R., Chen, K-U., Utilization of Isoflavones in Soybeans for Women with Menopausal Syndrome: An Overview, *Int J Mol Sci*, 2022. https://pubmed.ncbi.nlm.nih.gov/33809928/

49 Johnson S.A., Figueroa A., Navaei N., Wong A., Kalfon R., et al., Daily Blueberry Consumption Improves Blood Pressure and Arterial Stiffness in Postmenopausal Women with Pre- and Stage 1-hypertension: A Randomized, Double-blind, Placebo-controlled Clinical trial, *J Acad Nutr Diet*, 2015. https://pubmed.ncbi.nlm.nih.gov/25578927/

50 Khine W.W.T., Haldar S., De Loi S., et al., A Single Serving of Mixed Spices Alters Gut Microflora Composition: A Dose–Response Randomised Trial, *Sci Rep 11*, 2021. https://doi.org/10.1038/s41598-021-90453-7

51 Omagari K., Sakaki M., Tsujimoto Y., Shiogama Y., Iwanaga A., Ishimoto M., Yamaguchi A., Masuzumi M., Kawase M., Ichimura M., Yoshitake T., Miyahara Y., Coffee Consumption is Inversely Associated With Depressive Status in Japanese Patients with Type 2 Diabetes, *J Clin Biochem Nutr*, 2014. https://pubmed.ncbi.nlm.nih.gov/25320461/

52 Han K., Bose S., Wang J.H., Kim B.S., Kim M.J., Kim E.J., Kim H., Contrasting Effects of Fresh and Fermented Kimchi Consumption on Gut Microbiota Composition and Gene Expression Related to Metabolic Syndrome in Obese Korean Women, *Mol Nutr Food Res*, 2015. https://pubmed.ncbi.nlm.nih.gov/25688926/

53 Li X., Hong J., Wang Y., Pei M., Wang L., Gong Z., Trimethylamine-N-Oxide Pathway: A Potential Target for the Treatment of MAFLD, *Front Mol Biosci*, 2021. https://www.frontiersin.org/articles/10.3389/fmolb.2021.733507/full

Index

Acknowledgements

Jane

Huge thanks to the 'Menopausal Massif' at Wild Artichokes for their support, wisdom and sense of fun (plus for putting up with my singing), Miss Miller, Jo Vickers, Heather Morris and Peri Sarah Cowell.

Also to Kate Whitaker and Annie Rigg for a fun shoot with amazing pictures and styling. Everyone at Kyle especially Judith and Helena for giving me this opportunity. To Katherine Stonehouse for getting the ball rolling, and Dr Fed for passing on her knowledge and making it accesible.

Finally my son David, who continues to cook brilliantly and still surprises me with what you can put in a wrap.

Federica

Thank you to my loving family and husband for supporting me throughout all of my work. Thank you to the wonderful women in my life who this book is for; my mother for being a brilliant role model, my friends who are my support network, and to my beautiful daughters for being the driving force behind my passion and zest for life.

Thank you to my clients who brighten up my week and who live these changes and encourage me to spread the word. Thank you to Lavina and Sam for contributing to this book and for being part of this movement to improve women's health for the menopause and beyond.

Thank you to Tim Spector for your support and advice. Thank you to my fellow ZOEntists, my Imperial College colleagues and especially to Dr Lucy McCann who has become my right hand in finishing so many scientific projects. Last but not least thanks to Helena Sutcliffe at Octopus Books who asked me to write this book and is a joy to work with, and to Georgie Wolfinden whose PR skills have helped make my science comms dreams a reality.

First published in Great Britain in 2023 by Kyle Books, an imprint of
Octopus Publishing Group Ltd
Carmelite House
50 Victoria Embankment
London EC4Y 0DZ

www.octopusbooks.co.uk

An Hachette UK Company
www.hachette.co.uk

ISBN 978-1-80419-143-9

Distributed in the US by
Hachette Book Group
1290 Avenue of the Americas
4th and 5th Floors
New York, NY 10104

Distributed in Canada by
Canadian Manda Group
664 Annette St.
Toronto, Ontario, Canada M6S 2C8

Publishing Director: Judith Hannam
Publisher: Jo Copestick
Commissioning Editor: Helena Sutcliffe
Copy Editor: Vicky Orchard
Design: Yasia Williams and Paul Palmer-Edwards
Photography: Kate Whitaker
Food & props stylist: Annie Rigg
Illlustrations: Paul Palmer-Edwards
Production: Allison Gonsalves

A CIP catalogue record for this book is available from the British Library.

Printed and bound in China

10 9 8 7 6 5 4 3 2 1

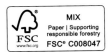